Global Advances in Wide Awake Hand Surgery

Editors

DONALD H. LALONDE
JIN BO TANG

HAND CLINICS

www.hand.theclinics.com

Consulting Editor
KEVIN C. CHUNG

February 2019 • Volume 35 • Number 1

ELSEVIER

1600 John F. Kennedy Boulevard • Suite 1800 • Philadelphia, Pennsylvania, 19103-2899

http://www.theclinics.com

HAND CLINICS Volume 35, Number 1
February 2019 ISSN 0749-0712, ISBN-13: 978-0-323-65457-9

Editor: Lauren Boyle
Developmental Editor: Kristen Helm

Hand Clinics (ISSN 0749-0712) is published quarterly by Elsevier Inc., 360 Park Avenue South, New York, NY 10010-1710. Months of publication are February, May, August, and November. Business and Editorial Offices: 1600 John F. Kennedy Blvd., Ste. 1800, Philadelphia, PA 19103-2899. Customer Service Office: 3251 Riverport Lane, Maryland Heights, MO 63043. Periodicals postage paid at New York, NY and at additional mailing offices. Subscription price is $435.00 per year (domestic individuals), $813.00 per year (domestic institutions), $100.00 per year (domestic students/residents), $501.00 per year (Canadian individuals), $947.00 per year (Canadian institutions), $546.00 per year (international individuals), $947.00 per year (international institutions), and $256.00 per year (international and Canadian students/residents). Foreign air speed delivery is included in all *Clinics* subscription prices. All prices are subject to change without notice. **POSTMASTER:** Send address changes to *Hand Clinics*, Elsevier Health Sciences Division, Subscription Customer Service, 3251 Riverport Lane, Maryland Heights, MO 63043. Customer Service (orders, claims, online, change of address): Elsevier Health Sciences Division, Subscription **Customer Service, 3251 Riverport Lane, Maryland Heights, MO 63043. Tel: 1-800-654-2452 (U.S. and Canada); 314-447-8871 (outside U.S. and Canada). Fax: 314-447-8029. E-mail: journalscustomerservice-usa@elsevier.com (for print support);** journalsonlinesupport-usa@elsevier.com (for online support).

Reprints. For copies of 100 or more of articles in this publication, please contact the Commercial Reprints Department, Elsevier Inc., 360 Park Avenue South, New York, New York 10010-1710. Tel.: 212-633-3874; Fax: 212-633-3820; E-mail: reprints@elsevier.com.

Hand Clinics is covered in *MEDLINE/PubMed (Index Medicus), Current Contents/Clinical Medicine, EMBASE/Excerpta Medica,* and *ISI/BIOMED.*

Contributors

CONSULTING EDITOR

KEVIN C. CHUNG, MD, MS
Chief of Hand Surgery, University of Michigan
Health System, Charles B.G. de Nancrede
Professor of Plastic Surgery and Orthopaedic
Surgery, Department of Surgery, Assistant
Dean for Faculty Affairs, Associate Director of
Global REACH, University of Michigan Medical
School, Ann Arbor, Michigan, USA

EDITORS

**DONALD H. LALONDE, BScHons, MSc, DSc,
MD, FRCSC**
Professor of Surgery, Division of Plastic
Surgery, Dalhousie University, Dalhousie
Medicine New Brunswick, Saint John, New
Brunswick, Canada

JIN BO TANG, MD
Professor and Chair, Department of Hand
Surgery, The Hand Surgery Research Center,
Affiliated Hospital of Nantong University,
Nantong, Jiangsu, China

AUTHORS

HEE CHAN AHN, MD
Director, W Institute for Hand & Reconstructive
Microsurgery, W General Hospital, Daegu, Korea

PETER C. AMADIO, MD
Dean for Research Academic Affairs, Lloyd A.
and Barbara A. Amundson Professor of
Orthopedics, Professor of Biomedical
Engineering, Department of Orthopedic
Surgery, Mayo Clinic, Rochester, Minnesota,
USA

**MOHAMMED SHOAIB ARSHAD, MBChB,
FRCS**
Fellow, Upper Limb Unit, Wrightington
Hospital, Wigan, Lancashire, United
Kingdom

EGEMEN AYHAN, MD
Attending Hand Surgeon, Hand Surgery,
Orthopaedics and Traumatology, University of
Health Sciences, Diskapi Yildirim Beyazit
Training and Research Hospital, Ankara,
Turkey

JAMES CHANG, MD
Division of Plastic and Reconstructive Surgery,
Johnson & Johnson Distinguished Professor of
Surgery (Plastic Surgery) & Orthopedic
Surgery, Stanford University Medical Center,
Palo Alto, California, USA

**DAFYDD S. EDWARDS, BSc(Hons), FRCS,
MD**
Fellow, Upper Limb Unit, Wrightington
Hospital, Wigan, Lancashire, United
Kingdom

VERENA J.M.M. FESTEN-SCHRIER, MD
Department of Orthopedic Surgery, Mayo
Clinic, Rochester, Minnesota, USA;
Department of Plastic, Reconstructive and
Hand Surgery, Erasmus Medical Center,
Rotterdam, The Netherlands

LIN LIN GAO, MD
Fellow, Chase Hand and Upper Limb Center,
Stanford University Medical Center, Palo Alto,
California, USA

KE TONG GONG, MD
Professor and Chair, Department of
Hand Surgery, Tianjin Hospital, Tianjin,
China

MICHAEL J. HAYTON, BSc(Hons), MBChB, FRCS
Consultant Orthopaedic Hand Surgeon,
Upper Limb Unit, Wrightington
Hospital, Wigan, Lancashire, United
Kingdom

SEBASTIAN HEDIGER, MD
Department of Hand Surgery, Bülach Hospital,
Diessenhofen, Switzerland

SIMON HUANG, FRCSEd (Plast)
Chirurgie Lindenpark, Surgical Day Case
Center, Kloten, Switzerland

CONSTANTINOS KRITIOTIS, MD, EBHS
Consultant, Orthopaedic Hand Surgeon,
Manchester Hand Centre, Salford Royal NHS
Foundation Trust, Manchester, United
Kingdom; Consultant, Orthopaedic Hand
Surgeon, Iasis Private Hospital, Paphos,
Cyprus

DONALD H. LALONDE, BScHons, MSc, DSc, MD, FRCSC
Professor of Surgery, Division of Plastic
Surgery, Dalhousie University, Dalhousie
Medicine New Brunswick, Saint John, New
Brunswick, Canada

BO LIU, MD, FRCS
Consultant Hand Surgeon, Department
of Hand Surgery, Beijing Ji Shui Tan
Hospital, Associate Professor, The 4th
Clinical Hospital of Peking University,
Beijing, China

AKBAR KHAN MOHAMMED, MS
Consultant Reconstructive Surgeon, Damien
Foundation Hospital, Nellore, Andhra Pradesh,
India

LINDSAY MUIR, MB, MChOrth, FRCS(Orth)
Consultant, Orthopaedic Hand Surgeon,
Manchester Hand Centre, Salford Royal
NHS Foundation Trust, Manchester,
United Kingdom; Orthopaedic Department,
Salford Royal Hospital, Salford, United
Kingdom

ZAFAR NAQUI, MBBS, FRCS (Orth)
Consultant, Orthopaedic Hand Surgeon,
Manchester Hand Centre, Salford Royal NHS
Foundation Trust, Manchester, United
Kingdom; Orthopaedic Department, Salford
Royal Hospital, Salford, United Kingdom

CHYE YEW NG, MBChB(Hons), FRCS, DipHandSurg (Br&Eur)
Consultant Hand and Peripheral Nerve
Surgeon, Upper Limb Unit, Wrightington
Hospital, Wigan, Lancashire, United
Kingdom

CHRISTIAN PETROPOLIS, MD, FRCSC
Attending Surgeon, Department of Plastic and
Reconstructive Surgery, University of
Manitoba, Winnipeg Health Sciences Centre,
Manitoba, Canada

ALISTAIR PHILLIPS, FRCS
Consultant, Orthopaedic Hand Surgeon,
Orthopaedic Department, University Hospital
Southampton NHS Foundation Trust,
Southampton General Hospital, Southampton,
United Kingdom

PEDRO JOSÉ PIRES NETO, MD
Hand Surgeon, Department of Orthopaedic
and Hand Surgery, Felício Rocho Hospital,
Belo Horizonte, Minas Gerais, Brazil

PETER CHARLES RHEE, DO, MS
Associate Professor, Department of
Orthopedic Surgery, Mayo Clinic, Rochester,
Minnesota, USA

SAMUEL RIBAK, MD, PhD
Head of the Hand Surgery Group,
Pontifical Catholic University of Campinas
(PUC-Campinas), Campinas, São Paulo,
Brazil

TRAJANO SARDENBERG, MD, PhD
Professor of Orthopaedics, Traumatology and
Hand Surgery, Department of Surgery and
Orthopedics, Botucatu Medical School, São
Paulo State University, UNESP, Botucatu, São
Paulo, Brazil

JIN BO TANG, MD
Professor and Chair, Department of Hand
Surgery, The Hand Surgery Research Center,
Affiliated Hospital of Nantong University,
Nantong, Jiangsu, China

MARGIE WHEELOCK, MD, FRCSC
Assistant Professor, Department of Plastic and
Reconstructive Surgery, Dalhousie University,
IWK Health Centre, Halifax, Nova Scotia,
Canada

SANG HYUN WOO, MD, PhD
President, W Institute for Hand &
Reconstructive Microsurgery, W General
Hospital, Daegu, Korea

SHU GUO XING, MD
Attending Surgeon, Department of
Hand Surgery, The Hand Surgery
Research Center, Affiliated Hospital of
Nantong University, Nantong, Jiangsu, China

JIAN HUA XU, MD
Attending Surgeon, Department of
Hand Surgery, Tianjin Hospital, Tianjin,
China

LU YI, MD
Attending Surgeon, Department of
Hand Surgery, Tianjin Hospital, Tianjin,
China

MYUNG JAE YOO, MD
Director, W Institute for Hand & Reconstructive
Microsurgery, W General Hospital, Daegu,
Korea

Contents

 Video content accompanies this article at http://www.hand.theclinics.com/.

> Injection of tumescent local anesthesia should no longer be painful. WALANT anesthesia, strong sutures, a slightly bulky repair, intraoperative testing of active movement, and judicious venting of the A2 and A4 pulleys improve results in flexor tendon repair. WALANT K wire finger fracture reduction permits intraoperative testing of K wire stability with active movement to facilitate early protected movement at 3 to 5 days after surgery. WALANT can decrease costs and garbage production while increasing accessibility and affordability. Several surgeons have found no infection difference when the K wires are inserted with full operating room sterility versus field sterility.

> This article summarizes the application of local anesthesia no tourniquet in 2 hand surgery centers in China, Nantong and Tianjin, where more than 12,000 patients were operated on with the new approach. This approach achieves excellent anesthetic and vasoconstrictive effects. In Nantong, surgeons performed fracture fixation, soft tissue tumor excision, and flap transfer in the hand with this approach. In Tianjin, surgeons applied it to cases of hand trauma emergency surgery. The authors' experience shows that this approach to hand surgery is safe, economical, and patient friendly, with no increase in infection rate.

> Wide-awake hand surgery is versatile and can be performed in a variety of settings for various pathologies. The benefits associated with wide-awake local anesthesia no tourniquet hand surgery can be extremely beneficial in the military health care system. Military medicine focuses on supporting soldiers in areas of combat, providing humanitarian care to local nationals, and to delivering health care to active duty soldiers and veterans in the domestic setting. The ability to perform hand

patient satisfaction rates. In both countries, patient education is a prerequisite for WALANT surgery. It increases the satisfaction rate among patients and enhances the patient-surgeon relationship. Patients need to know they can participate actively in a procedure, because a patient moving the hand during a procedure can improve the outcome.

has given surgeons the ability to visualize both static and dynamic movements of a joint, to show the pathology and discuss with the patient, and to visualize a patient's repaired structures. This reinforces confidence in surgeons and encourages patients to comply with postoperative rehabilitation.

Wide Awake surgery under Local Anesthesia with No Tourniquet (WALANT) has revolutionized clinical hand surgery, improving clinical outcomes and reducing post-operative pain and morbidity. It can also be used to deepen scientific knowledge, because the unsedated patient, with sensation intact and without the adverse effects of tourniquet neurapraxia or paralysis, can follow commands and actively move the limb after tendon and nerve surgery. These movements can be correlated with fingertip force, tendon tension, nerve conduction and amplitude, and muscle sarcomere length measurements to develop new insights into the effectiveness of many different tendon and nerve procedures in the hand.

The authors' experience demonstrates that wide-awake flap surgery in the hand is safe. The authors used this approach in 4 commonly used flaps in the hand in 27 patients: the extended Segmuller flap, the homo-digital reverse digital artery flap, the dorsal metacarpal artery perforator flap, and the Atasoy advancement flap. Wide-awake flap surgery works very well and safely achieved excellent anesthetic and vasoconstrictive effects in the authors' cases. The authors found that vasoconstriction caused by epinephrine mainly affects the capillaries and does not affect digital arteries and their major branches in the hand.

HAND CLINICS

ISSUE OF RELATED INTEREST:

Orthopedic Clinics of North America, January 2018 (Vol. 49, No. 1)
Outpatient Surgery
Michael J. Beebe, Clayton C. Bettin, James H. Calandruccio, Benjamin J. Grear,
Benjamin M. Mauck, William M. Mihalko, Jeffrey R. Sawyer, Thomas (Quin) Throckmorton,
Patrick C. Toy, and John C. Weinlein, *Editors*
Available at http://www.orthopedic.theclinics.com/

THE CLINICS ARE AVAILABLE ONLINE!
Access your subscription at:
www.theclinics.com

Preface

How the Wide Awake Tourniquet-Free Approach Is Changing Hand Surgery in Most Countries of the World

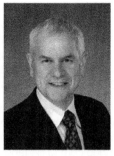 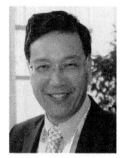

Donald H. Lalonde, MD   Jin Bo Tang, MD

Editors

Wide Awake Local Anesthesia No Tourniquet (WALANT) hand surgery has greatly increased in popularity and scope in the last 10 years. In 2018, there are surgeons in most countries of the world who apply this technique for at least some of their procedures. Wide awake hand surgery is performed without a tourniquet; only lidocaine with epinephrine is injected in the area where any dissection or painful manipulation of bones or Kirschner wires could cause pain.

In 2018, local anesthesia can be injected in a minimally painful fashion so that no sedation is required. Hand surgery can now be performed with the reduced costs, increased patient convenience, and simplicity of a tooth procedure in a dentist's office. The increased safety of eliminating all the risks of sedation and general anesthesia is appealing.

The simplification of hand surgery is having a profound effect on decreasing its cost and increasing its availability to the poor. Evidence-based sterility is enabling the performance of hand surgery outside of the main operating room, full sterility environment. Many simple procedures such as carpal tunnel surgery and trigger finger release can safely be performed in minor procedure rooms and in surgeons' offices. The decreased waste of unnecessary main operating room sterility material is contributing to the greening of surgery.

"Global Advances in Wide Awake Hand Surgery" explores some of the changes generated by WALANT around the world. The articles in this issue cover the latest innovations in sedation-free tourniquet-free surgery, which include almost zero pain with local anesthetic injection, better results in flexor tendon and finger fracture surgery, and wide awake fingertip flap reconstruction. Tendon transfers and their increased availability in leprosy patients are described. Hurdles and obstacles to the development of the technique as well as solutions and implementation all around the world are explored. The latest ideas that improve the patient's experience of hand surgery are described. Some authors provide current and future examples of WALANT as a research tool to increase our understanding of basic science physiology as well as provide improvements in hand surgery and therapy.

We would like to sincerely thank all of our hand surgeon authors from Brazil, Canada, China, Cyprus, England, India, Korea, Switzerland, Turkey, and the United States, who have produced great articles to show how WALANT is improving hand surgery for surgeons and their patients in their countries. We are also very grateful to our wonderful colleagues at Elsevier who have made this possible.

Donald H. Lalonde, MD
Dalhousie University
Suite C204
600 Main Street
Saint John, New Brunswick E2K 1J5, Canada

Jin Bo Tang, MD
Department of Hand Surgery
The Hand Surgery Research Center
Affiliated Hospital of Nantong University
20 West Temple Road
Nantong 226001, Jiangsu, China

E-mail addresses:
drdonlalonde@nb.aibn.com
dlalonde@drlalonde.ca (D.H. Lalonde)
jinbotang@yahoo.com (J.B. Tang)

Local Anesthesia Without Tourniquet in Hand and Forearm Surgery: My Story of Using and Promoting it

I am a fan of wide-awake hand surgery, and so are my colleagues. We are now using this technique for about one-fourth of our yearly 4000 to 5000 operations. In this editorial, I will walk you through my story and describe the major transitions that my colleagues and I have had in adopting this approach.

UNDERSTANDING THE UNIQUE ASPECTS: 2008

At the reception of the American Society for Surgery of the Hand (ASSH) meeting in Chicago in 2008, Don Lalonde and I met for the first time. I was with three of my colleagues from Nantong when Don introduced himself: "I come from Canada. Do you do hand surgery under local anesthesia with the patient wide awake?" Please note that Don did not mention epinephrine in this first conversation with me. I replied, "Yes, I do. In China, almost all hand surgery procedures are done with the patient wide awake because we use brachial plexus block without sedation in almost all of our patients. For minor procedures such as trigger finger and tissue coverage in fingertips, we all use local anesthesia in the hand or finger." My three colleagues were in this conversation. They also wondered why Dr Lalonde was asking about such a common technique. I do not remember whether Don said he used epinephrine or did not use the tourniquet. I left with the impression that Don was a nice, friendly Canadian hand surgeon, who wanted us to use wide-awake surgery. We were already using wide-awake surgery as our patients were not sedated, and they were always awake. The kindness of Don left me with greater impression than the surgery he talked about. In 2008 and 2009, my colleagues and I did not change anything we were doing because of the first conversation.

THE USE IN MY DEPARTMENT: 2010 TO 2014

After 2010, we noticed that Don spoke often in symposia to popularize the wide-awake approach. He presented at the ASSH meeting and frequently published on this topic in journals. His papers and talks attracted attention of one young colleague in my department, Dr Shu Guo Xing. In his late twenties at that time, Dr Xing, working in the group of Dr Ren Guo Xie, started to perform wide-awake hand surgery exactly as Don wrote and talked about in treating carpal tunnel releases, soft tissue resection, and fractures of the phalanges and metacarpals. In this period, we came to realize that it is better to try to introduce Chinese hand surgeons to this technique with the term "local anesthesia without tourniquet" (LANT) when introducing this method. The innovative components of the technique of Don's methods for Chinese surgeons are the elimination of the tourniquet with the use of tumescent local anesthesia with epinephrine for vasoconstriction. The words "wide awake" are not innovative to a country of surgeons who generally do not use sedation and commonly use local anesthetic nerve blocks to do hand surgery.

My friendship and communication with Don deepened in that period. I told all my colleagues in the department that we all should do this wide-awake surgery. I personally began to use it in carpal tunnel release, soft tissue tumor resection, tendon repair, and tenolysis. By 2011, the wide-awake surgery described by Don was nothing strange to all the surgeons in our department, although the use was not as widespread as it is now. In a pre-congress of the International Federation of Societies for Surgery of the Hand (IFSSH) meeting in 2011, Don visited Nantong for less than 24 hours, but we had wonderful time. In his usual way, he kept advocating this approach to all who attended this pre-congress in the morning, heading to airport with a lunch box.

GETTING THE MESSAGE TO OTHER UNITS AND URGING THEM TO ADOPT: FROM 2015

My colleagues and I became very fond of this approach and now use it routinely whenever the patients agree to this form of anesthesia. Since 2015, my major concern has been how to rapidly spread this approach to other units in China. I knew if I introduced "wide awake" to Chinese colleagues, they would not be interested because it would sound like something we had already been doing

Hand Clin 35 (2019) xv–xx
https://doi.org/10.1016/j.hcl.2018.10.002
0749-0712/19/© 2018 Published by Elsevier Inc.

daily for decades and by generations of hand surgeons. I therefore chose the approach of eliminating the words "wide awake." I emphasized that this was local anesthesia with epinephrine vasoconstriction with *no* tourniquet. Chinese hand surgeons realized this new form of wide-awake surgery was quite different from the "wide awake" they had previously used. The term "local anesthesia without tourniquet (LANT)" was much more meaningful to Chinese hand surgeons.

In 2015, I organized a LANT symposium at the annual Jixia Hand Surgery Forum. The first symposium on WALANT organized by Don was at the American Association for Hand Surgery meeting in 2016. The Jixia Forum was organized by the newly founded Association of Chinese-speaking Hand Surgery United, currently an IFSSH member. This yearly LANT symposium now attracts many attendees and has spread wide-awake hand surgery quickly in parts of China. I often hear from attendees: "I am using it now because I attended the symposium last year." At least 150 hand surgeons regularly use this approach in their practice because of these symposia. I have a burden of popularizing this approach in China, as it has a population greater than many countries together. The impact of this approach would be remarkable.

THE CHANGES IN SETUP IN MY DEPARTMENT: 2015 TO 2017

I have been thinking about how to incorporate LANT surgery in our departmental setup and improve the efficiency of our surgeons since 2015. Our department has 14 hand surgeons and 14 to 15 trainees, but our number of operation rooms was insufficient to accommodate such a large number of surgeons. Waiting for anesthesiologists was also an inefficient use of our surgical time.

Our hospital is always incredibly supportive of our hand surgery team! With the generous support from our institution, I converted and designated a small classroom inside the department to become a LANT operating room. We designed it to incorporate all that is necessary for any advanced LANT procedures (**Fig. 1**). It is a normal operating room with advanced lighting and airflow system, rather than a minor procedure room. The renovation took about a year. In 2017, this operating room started to function fully. We have one nurse who deals with sterilization and equipment and serves as a circulating nurse during surgery. This room easily accommodates 5 to 7 procedures per day under LANT. This operating room is only 5 to 20 meters from the academic offices of the surgeons, which is a remarkable time saver. In addition, we use existing ward staff, and therefore, no added

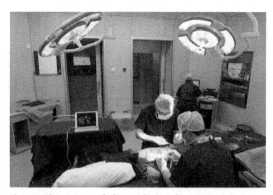

Fig. 1. The setup of the wide-awake operating room in the hospital of Nantong University. Two surgeons are operating on a patient, with one nurse circulating, while the patient is watching a movie using a tablet.

personnel are needed. With our new operating facility, our surgeons are now able to finish their cases before evening. The quality of life of both the patients and the surgeons is therefore improved. There is also a great cost saving for our system.

This operating room inside our department of hand surgery has attracted visitors from several different hospitals in China. Our model of an independent wide-awake operating room inside the department is spreading.

IN THE JIXIA HAND SURGERY FORUM IN CHINA IN 2018

The most recent wide-awake hand surgery symposium in China was in June 2018 (**Fig. 2**). Two things were quite impressive to me. First, among the hospitals where wide-awake surgery was routine, Tianjin Hospital impressed me with their vast number of patients. Dr Ke Tong Gong and his colleagues reported the use of this approach in 7600 patients in only 25 months. Dr Gong's department routinely carefully collects and documents each patient's information and the details of all procedures. They are collecting a large data bank of information on all categories of wide-awake hand surgery. For example, they have documented treatment of closed ruptures of the tendons in 45 patients, 110 cubital tunnel releases, and 340 patients with open reduction and internal fracture fixation. They have not yet written about this as they are usually too busy to report their extensive experience in individual categories of surgery, although this issue of *Hand Clinics* includes a review of their experience. Their way of recording patient and procedure information and archiving them appears to be an efficient way to document wide-awake cases.

Second, a conversation with a hand surgeon impressed me. He approached me during one of

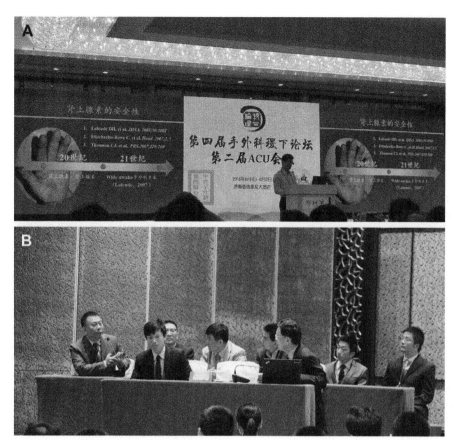

Fig. 2. Symposiums on LANT hand surgery in China. (*A*) The most recent symposium on June 1, 2018 organized by the Association of Chinese-speaking Hand Surgeon United through its meeting and Jixia Forum. (*B*) Panelists in a symposium on LANT in Nantong on June 4, 2016. Front row, from right to left: Jin Bo Tang and Shu Guo Xing. Back row, center: Ke Tong Gong. Zhang Jun Pan, Xiang Zhou, Jun Tan and Zeng Tao Wang are in the back row.

the breaks and said to me: "Dr Tang, I thought 'wide-awake' hand surgery is something new, but after listening to today's talks by these people, it is not new. We have done this in hand cases for a long time. We do not use a tourniquet, we never put patients to sleep, and we use local anesthesia." Then I asked him: "Do you use epinephrine?" He answered: "Yes, we do. We mix epinephrine in saline. We press gauzes soaked with saline-diluted epinephrine over the tissues after we make surgical incisions or when we treat open injuries of the hand and fingers. We have known for a long time that epinephrine can be used in the hand and fingers without risk, and a high concentration of epinephrine does no harm as well." He further explained that "we call saline with epinephrine *"blood-stopping liquid."* This is pronounced in Chinese as "zhi-xue-ye." Zhi means stopping; xue means blood, and ye means liquid. I said to him: "It makes sense that you use fluid to stop bleeding in an operating field. You have already been doing this type of surgery

for many years? Why you did not popularize it to all over China or all over the world? If you have had done so, you would be Don Lalonde." He left me when the sessions restarted. I regretted that I did not write down his name. Later, I asked a colleague if he could help me locate that surgeon. The colleague informed me that many hand surgeons in the central part of China use "blood-stopping liquid" regularly, and it is not necessary to look for any one surgeon who is using this approach to avoid the tourniquet.

China is a vast country. New knowledge of old practices in distant parts of the country is not surprising. I live in Nantong. It is a medium-sized city in China, but its population is more than that of Finland. Just as it is not surprising that a surgeon in one European country does not know what is done in another country, we are not surprised to learn of many unknown different practices in other parts of China. I was very impressed that some surgeons in some parts of China already use epinephrine extensively in hands and fingers to operate without a tourniquet. It supplies another explanation for why Chinese surgeons have so quickly and easily adopted Don Lalonde's approach of using epinephrine. For those surgeons in other regions of the world who still are hesitant to use epinephrine in the hand and fingers, the above message should help.

The unexpected Chinese use of "blood-stopping fluid" further corroborates the wisdom of the long-standing practice of epinephrine injection into fingers and the hand in Canada. It remains to be seen whether topical "blood-stopping fluid" works better or worse than injected epinephrine in standard WALANT surgery. Perhaps "blood-stopping fluid" has advantages in deeper tissues where injected epinephrine does not reach.

PUSHING THE LIMIT OF LANT SURGERY: TWO CHALLENGES TO MY PRACTICE

In the last two years, my colleagues and I have explored the limits of LANT surgery. It came to me that flap surgery can be safely performed with LANT with epinephrine use. I have been regularly using epinephrine in any V-Y or advancement flap transfer in fingers or thumbs (**Fig. 3**). Drs Shu Guo Xing and Tian Mao have expanded this method to extended V-Y flaps and pedicled perforator flap transfers in the hand and fingers. We now consider that any ordinary pedicled flap can be harvested under LANT. Harvesting a perforator flap should perhaps be approached with more caution.

The feasibility of extensive bony surgery under LANT has been a question for me and my colleagues for years. We read that fusion of the finger joints and thumb basal joint surgery can be done with LANT. However, we remained uncertain about the possibility of surgery involving stripping periosteum and osteotomy in the midshaft of a phalanx or metacarpal. However, in the past two years, we have regularly performed benign tumor excision from phalanges or metacarpals, stripped periosteum, chiseled bone, and even bone grafts (**Fig. 4**). We have done it all with the patient not feeling any pain at all. They only feel the first injection of anesthetic mixture and then pressure in the bones during the operation.

Our recent experience with LANT leads us to consider that this technique can be used for most patients with nondevastating hand disorders if the patient is willing to have it. If we can use LANT in flap harvest with *safety* and in removing bone tumors *without pain*, I cannot think of any procedures in which we cannot use this technique. Two possible remaining contraindications to the use of LANT may be infection in the operative site and the unwillingness of surgeons to use it.

THE KEYS TO POPULARIZE IT ARE OUR UNDERSTANDING AND WILLINGNESS OF ADOPT IT

Some surgeons may complain that the patients do not want to be wide awake. It is true some patients may not like it. That is why more than half of our procedures on patients are still not done with LANT. Some surgeons still prefer a truly bloodless field when dissecting deep tissues or the when surgery is truly extensive. However, it is important that surgeons present the LANT option to their patients in a positive light and make them aware of its benefits. In many cases, it is the surgeons who do not want to do it when they say that the patients do not want this approach. Should the surgeon present a fair and honest comparative discussion of risks and benefits of LANT versus traditional hand surgery anesthesia, many patients would choose LANT. Keeping patients blind to the advantages of this novel approach would deny them the opportunity to benefit from it. Therefore, it is our responsibility as surgeons to present this choice to the patient. The key to popularizing it is our willingness to understand its benefits and adopt it.

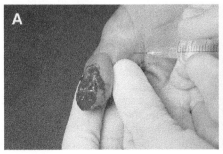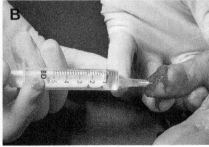

Fig. 3. Injection of local anesthetics with epinephrine into the (*A*) digital nerve and (*B*) fingertip for local advancement flaps is safe.

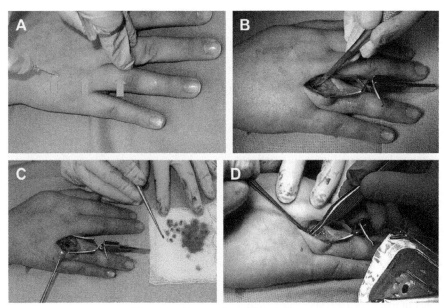

Fig. 4. Osteochondroma removal and bone grafting under wide-awake setting. (*A*) The sites of injection of local anesthesia, 1% lidocaine with 1:100,000 epinephrine. (*B*) A longitudinal extensor tendon splinting incision and a window made on the dorsal phalangeal cortex with a chisel. (*C*) Osteochondroma was removed. (*D*) Bone grafting.

TEACHING IS IMPORTANT, AND INCORPORATING SCIENCE INTO A CLINICAL TECHNIQUE IS NECESSARY

I was very impressed by Don for his way of "teaching." I remember he said on several occasions: "Let's teach them how to do." I feel this is a very positive and straightforward way to popularize a new technique. Don has been tireless in teaching this approach. He is usually willing to give any number of talks to the audience to popularize this technique as well as tendon repair, treatment of fractures, and so forth, in his own words "for the patients." As Don has written in his article in this issue of *Hand Clinics*, the use of epinephrine in hand surgery to achieve a less-bleeding operating field has been a practice in Canada for several decades. However, it is Don who brought it to worldwide attention and carried out a series of clinical studies to define this procedure. This is a vivid example of how popularizing a technique is impactful and how scientifically defining and refining a clinical technique is important. Clearly, Don brought science to this procedure and got the message to as many surgeons as he could with his tireless traveling, talks, and demonstrations. He has been in as many countries in the world as he could possibly go. I was very privileged to meet him and discuss with him frequently.

As a great friend of Don with frequent communication, I understand very deeply his passion to popularize this technique, his desire to help patients, and his enthusiasm in communicating with colleagues of all levels.

SUMMARY

A few key points about the WALANT or LANT technique and its popularization are as follows:

1. Wide-awake hand surgery, as it is known in North America, is in fact a procedure of local anesthesia without sedation and with no tourniquet use, but with the use of epinephrine to decrease bleeding during surgery.
2. In many countries, patients are not usually sedated. The term LANT (local anesthesia no tourniquet) may therefore be more meaningful to all hand surgeons regardless of region.
3. The use of epinephrine in the fingers, thumbs, and hand is certainly safe. It achieves a relatively bloodless field, rather than absolutely bloodless field. Epinephrine hemostasis is usually adequate for good hand surgery.
4. The maximal effect of stopping bleeding occurs by 25 minutes after injection[1] and can last for 4 to 5 hours, but surgeons do not necessarily need to wait 25 minutes to start the surgery. By 5 to 10 minutes after injection, there is enough of a decrease in bleeding to accommodate dissection and repair very well.
5. Modern techniques of local anesthesia delivery can greatly reduce anesthetic pain. Good technique results in the patient feeling no pain

except for the first poke of a very fine needle despite very commonly feeling pressure or traction of the tissues. With more recent injection techniques, even the initial needle poke can be pain free.[2]

6. LANT can be used in most hand surgery procedures from carpal tunnel release to flap transfer.[3–8] Surgery in the bone can be performed with this approach.[9]

7. The major benefit of LANT in improving the quality of reparative procedure is that patients can move their digits and hand during surgery to ensure that the repairs of tendons, bones, and joints are sufficiently strong, are properly tensioned, and move well.

8. LANT has been popularized very rapidly, but further promotion of this valuable technique is necessary. Surgeons should be open to this technique and present it to their patients in the decision-making process.

9. The benefits of this approach should be recognized beyond the saving of medical costs and rapid recovery.[9,10] Its impact on a surgeon's quality of life and hospital resources should be considered. All hand surgeons should seriously consider LANT for the benefit of their patients and their hand surgery service.

Jin Bo Tang, MD
Department of Hand Surgery
The Hand Surgery Research Center
Affiliated Hospital of Nantong University
Nantong 226001, Jiangsu, China

E-mail address:
jinbotang@yahoo.com

REFERENCES

1. Mckee DE, Lalonde DH, Thoma A, et al. Achieving the optimal epinephrine effect in wide awake hand surgery using local anesthesia without a tourniquet. Hand (N Y) 2015;10:613–5.
2. Lalonde DH. Conceptual origins, current practice, and views of wide awake hand surgery. J Hand Surg Eur Vol 2017;42:886–95.
3. Lalonde DH. "Hole-in-one" local anesthesia for wide-awake carpal tunnel surgery. Plast Reconstr Surg 2010;126:1642–4.
4. Lalonde DH. Wide-awake flexor tendon repair. Plast Reconstr Surg 2009;123:623–5.
5. Tang JB. Wide-awake primary flexor tendon repair, tenolysis, and tendon transfer. Clin Orthop Surg 2015;7:275–81.
6. Wong J, Lin CH, Chang NJ, et al. Digital revascularization and replantation using the wide-awake hand surgery technique. J Hand Surg Eur Vol 2017;42: 621–5.
7. Xing SG, Mao T. The use of local anaesthesia with epinephrine in the harvest and transfer of an extended Segmuller flap in the fingers. J Hand Surg Eur Vol 2018;43:783–4.
8. Xing SG, Mao T. Temporary tourniquet use after epinephrine injection to expedite wide awake emergency hand surgeries. J Hand Surg Eur Vol 2018;43: 888–9.
9. Tang JB, Gong KT, Zhu L, et al. Performing hand surgery under local anesthesia without a tourniquet in China. Hand Clin 2017;33:415–24.
10. Gong KT, Xing SG. How to establish and standardize wide-awake hand surgery: experience from China. J Hand Surg Eur Vol 2017;42: 868–70.

Latest Advances in Wide Awake Hand Surgery

Donald H. Lalonde, MSc, DSc, MD, FRCSC

KEYWORDS

- WALANT • Finger epinephrine • Wide awake surgery • No tourniquet hand surgery
- Sedation-free hand surgery • Tumescent local anesthesia

KEY POINTS

- The injection of tumescent local anesthesia should no longer be painful in 2018.
- Wide awake local anesthesia no tourniquet (WALANT) anesthesia, strong sutures, a slightly bulky repair, intraoperative testing of active movement, and judicious venting of the A2 and A4 pulleys have improved results in flexor tendon repair surgery.
- WALANT K wire finger fracture reduction permits intraoperative testing of K wire stability with active movement to facilitate early protected movement at 3 to 5 days after surgery.
- There is increasing evidence that WALANT decreases costs and garbage production while increasing accessibility and affordability of hand surgery.

 Video content accompanies this article at http://www.hand.theclinics.com/.

INTRODUCTION

Traditional hand surgery is performed with a tourniquet to create a bloodless field. Tourniquet pain creates a need for sedation in most countries. Evidence based medicine has proven that epinephrine vasoconstriction is safe in the finger, especially with the advent of phentolamine rescue.[1–4] This has eliminated the need for the tourniquet for most hand surgery because visibility with epinephrine vasoconstriction is very acceptable.[5]

Most hand operations can be performed with WALANT today.[6] The year 2016 saw the first English book published on the surject of wide awake hand surgery,[7] followed by the Chinese version publication in 2017.[8] Although it has been performed in Canada for over 40 years, WALANT has rapidly gained popularity in the rest of the world in less than 10 years' time.

FOUR RECENT ADVANCES

The Injection of Tumescent Local Anesthesia for Hand Surgery Should No Longer Be Painful in 2018

It is now known that tumescent local anesthesia with lidocaine and epinephrine can be injected in an almost pain-free fashion over large areas such as the whole hand, wrist, and forearm.[9–12] Minimal pain local anesthesia injection can be easily and reliably taught to medical students and residents,[13] so all surgeons can readily pick up this simple technical skill. This section of the article will detail and show in video how large areas of

Disclosure Statement: D.H. Lalonde is the editor of the book Wide Awake Hand Surgery (Thieme Publishers), published in 2016. He makes no profit on the sales of the book. All royalties go to the American Association for Hand Surgery Lean and Green effort, which is dedicated to decreasing unnecessary cost and garbage production in hand surgery.
Division of Plastic Surgery, Dalhousie University, Dalhousie Medicine New Brunswick, Suite C204, 600 Main Street, Saint John, New Brunswick E2K 1J5, Canada
E-mail address: dlalonde@drlalonde.ca

Hand Clin 35 (2019) 1–6
https://doi.org/10.1016/j.hcl.2018.08.002
0749-0712/19/© 2018 Elsevier Inc. All rights reserved.

the hand, wrist, and forearm can be anesthetized with the patient only feeling the initial poke of a 27 gauge needle for pain.

There are still many surgeons who hurt patients unnecessarily when they inject local anesthesia, because they are unaware of these advances. That pain drives them to need sedation for their surgery. The recipe and video, as well as the referenced papers and their on-line videos, eliminate this need for sedation.

When using sharp needles for injection, several small technical details decrease the pain of injection:

1. Use finer needles such as 27 gauge (0.41 mm) routinely for injection, because they hurt less and force a slower less painful injection.
2. Buffer the lidocaine and epinephrine with 8.4% bicarbonate at a ratio of 10 mL to 1 mL to decrease the pain of acidic local anesthetic solution.
3. Stabilize the syringe with 2 hands so the patient does not feel painful needle movement before the needle site is numb.
4. Insert the needle perpendicular to the skin, because it hurts more to insert the needle parallel to the skin.
5. Push the skin into the needle instead of pushing the needle into the skin. The sensory noise of mild pinch, movement, and pressure at the needle entry site decreases the pain of the first poke.
6. Inject at least 2 to 10 mL just underneath the skin (not in the skin) without moving the needle at all. Let the local anesthesia diffuse into the tissues without moving the sharp needle into live anesthetized nerves.
7. Always inject antegrade and have at least 1 to 2 cm of local anesthesia ahead of the slowly advancing sharp needle tip. Do not move the needle much. Put in the volume and let the local anesthetic diffuse into the tissues without risking sharp needle advancement pain.
8. When injecting large areas, reinsert the needle inside 1 cm of the border of areas that are clearly numbed with evident white epinephrine vasoconstriction. Never reinsert the needle into an area that is not solidly numb.
9. Always err on too much local solution instead of not enough. The only exception is in the fingers, where 2 mL on the volar side and 2 mL on the dorsal side of the proximal and middle phalanges are sufficient.
10. The goal is to have visible and palpable local anesthetic under the skin 2 cm beyond anywhere the surgeon is going to cut, dissect, or manipulate broken bones.
11. Always score yourself with patient feedback during the injection process. Ask the patient to tell you every time he or she feels any pain while you are injecting. To get better, you need to know how often you hurt a patient during each injection. This is the best way the injector can improve his or her skills as a painless injector. The goal of a good injector is to have the patient only feel pain once on the first poke, and then no more pain at all.
12. A good injector never needs additional local anesthesia to top up areas that are sore during the procedure because of an inadequate volume of local anesthetic in the initial injection. Top ups should be avoided just as good anesthesiologists avoid inadvertently waking patients up during general anesthesia.
13. Use blunt-tipped filler cannulas for injection of large areas such as forearm tendon transfers.

Cannula injection of local anesthesia

A new advance in decreasing the pain of injection of tumescent local anesthesia over large areas was first published in 2014.[14] Fine 25 and 27 gauge blunt-tipped cannulas[15] can now pass through subcutaneous fat without pain to facilitate more rapid injection of large volumes of local anesthesia for procedures such as forearm tendon transfers. The skin is first anesthetized with small 27 or 30 gauge needles. Larger needles such as a 22 or 20 gauge needle make a hole in the skin through which a 25 or 27 gauge cannula is easily inserted. These 2 inch (5 cm) cannulas can then rapidly inject large volumes of tumescent local anesthesia to both the volar and dorsal forearm (Video 1).

Tumescent local anesthesia means enough local anesthesia that you can see it and feel it under the skin anywhere you might cause pain. It is like an extravascular Bier block but only where one needs it. Motor nerves are preserved so you can see active movement by a comfortable cooperative tourniquet free unsedated patient before you close the skin. You can make adjustments in your reconstruction as dictated by intraoperative active movement.

WALANT Anesthesia, Strong Sutures, a Slightly Bulky Repair, Intraoperative Testing of Active Movement and Judicious Venting of the A2 and A4 Pulleys Have Greatly Improved Results in Flexor Tendon Repair Surgery

One of the most important papers ever written in flexor tendon repair was published by Jin Bo Tang and colleagues[16] in 2017. In a series of 300 flexor tendon repairs by junior and mid-level

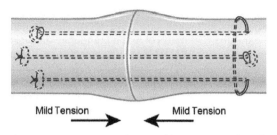

Fig. 1. A strong suture (6-strand looped suture) with 20% to 30% bunching of repair. This type of strong repair can be tested with intraoperative active movement with WALANT. The patient can prove this will not gap. The bulky repair will glide with a full range of motion with judicious pulley venting as described in the text. (*From* Tang JB, Zhou X, Pan ZJ, et al. Strong digital flexor tendon repair, extension-flexion test, and early active flexion: experience in 300 tendons. Hand Clin 2017;33(3):460; with permission.)

hand surgeons, there was only 1 rupture, and the range of motion results were over 80% excellent in 3 different centers following the same protocol. The essential features of this protocol are

1. A minimum of 0.7 to 1 cm purchase in both tendon stumps
2. Bulkiness of 10% to 30% at the repair site (**Fig. 1**)
3. A 6-strand M Tang repair (see **Fig. 1**)
4. Venting up to one-half of the A2 pulley or all of the A4 pulley if required, with never more than 2 cm of total pulley venting
5. Digital full-fist flexion and full-finger extension test during the surgery to make sure the repair does not gap and to ensure that it fits through remaining pulleys before skin closure
6. Up to half a fist of true active movement after passive warm up as part of the postoperative early protected movement program. This is not Kleinert rubber bands. This is not full fist place and hold. Essentially the same surgical and postoperative regimen is being used in Saint John[17,18] as Jin Bo Tang uses in China.[16]
7. The author would add a seventh important element to consistently get excellent results after flexor tendon repair. Use as much intraoperative time as possible to educate patients to avoid complications. The surgeon has the unsedated patient's full attention during the surgery. Instead of talking to the nurses about the weather, ask the patient what he or she originally was planning to do that week. During the procedure, the author explains to the patient how to avoid rupture. The author also explains that when that when the patient starts to move his or her hand at 3 to 5 days after surgery, he or she should be off all pain killers,

and can move the finger but cannot use it (Video 2).

Twenty percent of surveyed American hand surgeons have already performed WALANT flexor tendon repair despite the recent advent of the technique.[19] The great appeal of WALANT lies in the viewing of full-fist flexion and full-finger extension of a freshly repaired tendon. If there is gapping, which happens 7% of the time when the repair is not 30% bulky with tension,[20] one can fix it during surgery, so it does not rupture after surgery. If the repair does not easily glide through the pulleys, the surgeon can divide up to 2 cm of pulley, including all A4 and at least up to half of A2. This greatly decreases the need for tenolysis after flexor tendon repair. The surgeon knows that the repair will work before he or she closes the skin.

WALANT K Wire Finger Fracture Reduction Permits Intraoperative Testing of K Wire Stability with Active Movement to Facilitate Early Protected Movement at 3 to 5 Days After Surgery

Early protected movement after K wiring finger fractures is just as important as early protected movement after flexor tendon repair for the same reason; a still finger is a useless finger.

If K wired finger fractures are immobilized for 2 to 6 weeks, all gliding tendons and soft tissues adhere to the callus of the fracture and frequently result in permanent stiffness of finger joints, as occurs in prolonged immobilization of flexor tendon repairs. The author has been using early protective movement at 3 to 5 days in a controlled hand therapy environment after surgery for many years. The author is getting better results than when finger fractures were immobilized.[21,22]

Details of how to inject local anesthesia for WALANT K wiring have been published.[23] Lidocaine with epinephrine is injected proximal to distal so the patient only feels the proximal needle pokes. Both dorsal and volar distal hand and finger surfaces are injected, no more than 2 mL per phalanx on both the palmar and dorsal midline of the finger proximal and middle phalanges.

After K wire insertion, the comfortable tourniquet-free patient actively makes a full fist of flexion and full extension while the surgeon examines the stability of the fracture and K wires on the low power fluoroscope. If additional K wires are required to make the fracture functionally stable, they are inserted, and movement is tested again. If the fracture does not move with a full range of flexion and extension the day of surgery, it will not likely move with 30° of interphalangeal movement 4 days later.

For 3 to 5 days after surgery, the hand is elevated and immobilized to let the swelling come down and to get the patient off all pain medication. Collagen formation does not start until day 3.

As in WALANT flexor tendon surgery, some of the intraoperative time is used wisely to educate the patient on how he will be allowed to move the finger at 3 to 5 days after surgery under the supervision of hand therapists. The hand therapist is frequently invited into the minor procedure room during the K wire surgery so the patient can meet the therapist and establish him or her as part of the decision making team. The hand therapist will play a large role in the postoperative movement of these patients. He or she will build a splint. With the surgeon, he or she will educate the patient on the principles of pain guided therapy, pain-guided movement, and pain-guided healing.

Patients start to move the interphalangeal joints under the supervision of hand therapists. The key rule is that they must not do what hurts. The author encourages 30° of painless interphalangeal joint movement, which creates at least 5 mm of profundus gliding. If there is no painful movement, there will be few K wire infections. If there is no painful movement, the risk of losing a reduction will be small. The author removes the K wires when the fractures are no longer sore to palpation, which is clinical healing. Clinical healing will frequently be evident long before radiological healing in finger fractures. Radiological healing in finger fractures is not a useful sign for removal of K wires.

The author does not do early protected movement of K wired finger fractures in unstable fractures or in patients who are not cooperative or not able to be drug free for therapy. If they are on pain killers, they do not know what hurts (Video 3).

Increasing Evidence That WALANT Decreases Costs and Garbage Production While Increasing Accessibility and Affordability of Hand Surgery

Eliminating the need for sedation and the tourniquet has permitted moving many minor hand procedures such as carpal tunnel and trigger fingers out of the main operating room. Several recent papers have demonstrated that these major financial savings can be realized everywhere, including in American military hospitals.[24–28] Surgeons often lament that they cannot control costs of health care. In hand surgery, choosing WALANT enables surgeons to do it.

This volume of Hand Clinics explores the increasing use of WALANT in some developing countries. Many patients in many countries cannot afford hand surgery because of the high costs of sedation and main operating room sterility. Dr. Amir Adham Ahmada of Kuala Lumpur in Malaysia routinely uses WALANT for distal radius and ulna fracture plating.[29] The decrease in cost has greatly increased access to this type of operation in his patient population. He is among many surgeons who are now able to offer plating for forearm fracture surgery to less wealthy patients. Drs. Gilles Candelier and Thomas Apard are also routinely plating radius fractures with WALANT in France.

Dr. Akbar Khan from India has started leprosy surgery in India with WALANT. The paper describing his first 18 months of experience is part of this Hand Clinics volume. One of the great appealing factors in his patient population is the decreased cost and therefore increased availability of hand surgery for leprosy patients.

There is increasing evidence showing no difference in infection outcomes with field sterility (4 towels, gloves, mask) compared with full operating room sterility (gowns, drapes, and floor washing between cases) for simple hand surgery such as carpal tunnel. A prospective study of 6 surgeons in 5 cities with over 1500 cases of field sterility carpal tunnel yielded only 6 minor infections in which only 4 patients only received oral antibiotics.[30] There were no deep space infections requiring drainage and no hospitalizations for intravenous antibiotics. The move to a lean and green decrease in garbage generated from hand surgery could be enormous if all hospitals and surgery centers moved to field sterility for carpal tunnel and trigger fingers.[24]

Roughly half of Canadian hospitals have moved K wire insertion out of the main operating room and into the field sterility environment of minor procedure rooms where skin cancers are excised. Several surgeons with large volumes of experience of inserting K wires for finger fracture have found no infection difference when the K wires are inserted with full operating room sterility versus field sterility (4 towels, gloves, mask, outside the main operating room in minor procedure rooms).There currently are 10 Canadian hospitals across the country participating in a prospective study comparing infection rates with K wire insertion with field sterility versus full main operating room sterility. In the first 150 of 1000 cases, there is no difference in infection rates.

Moving hand fractures and tendon repairs out of the main operating room and into the clinic minor procedure rooms has meant a great decrease of night work for a lot of hand trauma surgeries in Canada. These cases are now performed Monday to Friday in the daytime at the surgeon's convenience in many centers such as Saint John,

Calgary, and Ottawa now. The need for main operating room time and anesthesiologist availability has been eliminated in these centers. The author feels that performing this type of surgery is better when surgeons are well rested in daytime hours.

NEW WALANT WEB SITE

Dr. Alistair Phillips of England has spent the better part of a year launching a new educational interaction Web site for surgeons and hand therapists on the whole topic of WALANT. The Web site launched on March 16, 2018. For those who would like more information, papers, videos, or advice on WALANT surgery, please visit https://walant.surgery/.[31]

SUMMARY

WALANT surgery is rapidly growing in most countries throughout the world. WALANT courses have been offered in China, the United States, Canada, Mexico, Brazil, Venezuela, Columbia, Iceland, Sweden, Italy, France, England, Germany, England, Hungary, Georgia, India, Dubai, Khatar, Indonesia, Malaysia, Philippines, Japan, Australia, New Zealand, Ghana, South Africa, Malawi, Marocco, and the Bahamas. There are now surgeons in all of those countries and more who are performing some form of WALANT surgery on a regular basis.

The reasons for the rapid increase in popularity include increased patient convenience, satisfaction, and safety. In addition, the surgery is much less costly and more environmentally friendly. Surgeons can get better results when they can see intraoperative comfortable active movement in operations like tendon and fracture surgery. Intraoperative education of the patient to decrease complications is another major bonus.

SUPPLEMENTARY DATA

Supplementary data related to this article can be found online at https://doi.org/10.1016/j.hcl.2018.08.002.

REFERENCES

1. Nodwell T, Lalonde DH. Howlong does it take phentolamine to reverse adrenaline-induced vasoconstriction in the finger and hand? A prospective randomized blinded study: the Dalhousie project experimental phase. Can J Plast Surg 2003;11:187.
2. Lalonde DH, Bell M, Benoit P, et al. A multicenter prospective study of 3110 consecutive cases of elective epinephrine use in the fingers and hand: the Dalhousie Project clinical phase. J Hand Surg Am 2005;30:1061.
3. Fitzcharles-Bowe C, Denkler KA, Lalonde DH. Finger injection with high-dose (1:1000) epinephrine: does it cause finger necrosis and should it be treated? Hand (N Y) 2007;2:5.
4. Thomson CJ, Lalonde DH, Denkler KA. A critical look at the evidence for and against elective epinephrine use in the finger. Plast Reconstr Surg 2007;119:260.
5. McKee DE, Lalonde DH, Thoma A, et al. Achieving the optimal epinephrine effect in wide awake hand surgery using local anesthesia without a tourniquet. Hand (N Y) 2015;10:613–5.
6. Lalonde DH, Wong A. Dosage of local anesthesia in wide awake hand surgery. J Hand Surg Am 2013;38:2025–8.
7. Lalonde DH. Wide awake hand surgery. New York: Thieme; 2016.
8. Tang JB. Wide awake hand surgery. Shanghai (China): Shanghai Scientific & Technical Publishers; 2017.
9. Strazar AR, Leynes PG, Lalonde DH. Minimizing the pain of local anesthesia injection. Plast Reconstr Surg 2013;132:675–84.
10. Lalonde DH. "Hole-in-one" local anesthesia for wide awake carpal tunnel surgery. Plast Reconstr Surg 2010;126:1642–4.
11. Lalonde DH, Jagodzinski N, Phillips A. How to inject local anaesthesia with minimal pain. In: Lalonde DH, editor. Wide awake hand surgery. New York: Thieme; 2016. p. 37–48.
12. Lalonde DH. Safe epinephrine in the finger means no tourniquet. In: Lalonde DH, editor. Wide awake hand surgery. New York: Thieme; 2016. p. 37.
13. Farhangkhoee H, Lalonde J, Lalonde DH. Teaching medical students and residents how to inject local anesthesia almost painlessly. Can J Plast Surg 2012;20:169–72.
14. Lalonde D, Wong A. Local anesthetics: what's new in minimal pain injection and best evidence in pain control. Plast Reconstr Surg 2014;134:40S–9S.
15. Available at: https://cosmofrance.net/?gclid=EAIaIQobChMIyYKK5oip2QIVULbACh16bQG4EAAYASAAEgKzPfD_BwE. Accessed February 15, 2018.
16. Tang JB, Zhou X, Pan ZJ, et al. Strong digital flexor tendon repair, extension-flexion test, and early active flexion: experience in 300 tendons. Hand Clin 2017;33:455–63.
17. Lalonde DH, Higgins A. Wide awake flexor tendon repair in the finger. Plast Reconstr Surg Glob Open 2016;4:e797.
18. Lalonde DH, Higgins A. Flexor tendon repair postoperative rehabilitation: the Saint John protocol. Plast Reconstr Surg Glob Open 2016;4:e1134.
19. Gibson PD, Sobol GL, Ahmed IH. Zone II flexor tendon repairs in the United States: trends in current management. J Hand Surg Am 2017;42:e99–108.

20. Higgins A, Lalonde DH, Bell M, et al. Avoiding flexor tendon repair rupture with intraoperative total active movement examination. Plast Reconstr Surg 2010; 126:941–5.

21. Gregory S, Lalonde DH, Leung LT. Minimally invasive finger fracture management, wide-awake closed reduction, k-wire fixation and early protective movement. Hand Clin 2014;30:7–15.

22. Jones NF, Jupiter JB, Lalonde DH. Common fractures and dislocations of the hand. Plast Reconstr Surg 2012;130:722e.

23. Lalonde DH. Finger fractures. In: Lalonde DH,, editor. Wide awake hand surgery. New York: Thieme; 2016. p. 237.

24. Van Demark RE Jr, Smith VJ, Fiegen A. Lean and green hand surgery. J Hand Surg Am 2018;43:179–81.

25. Rhee PC, Fischer MM, Rhee LS, et al. Cost savings and patient experiences of a clinic-based, wide-awake hand surgery program at a Military Medical Center: a critical analysis of the first 100 procedures. J Hand Surg Am 2017;42:e139–47.

26. Chatterjee A1, McCarthy JE, Montagne SA, et al. A cost, profit, and efficiency analysis of performing carpal tunnel surgery in the operating room versus the clinic setting in the United States. Ann Plast Surg 2011;66:245–8.

27. Bismil MS, Bismil QM, Harding D, et al. Transition to total one-stop wide-awake hand surgery service audit: a retrospective review. JRSM Short Rep 2012;3:23.

28. Leblanc MR, Lalonde J, Lalonde DH. A detailed cost and efficiency analysis of performing carpal tunnel surgery in the main operating room versus the ambulatory setting in Canada. Hand (N Y) 2007;2: 173–8.

29. Amir AA, Mohammad AI. Plating of an isolated fracture of shaft of ulna under local anaesthesia and periosteal nerve block. Trauma Case Rep 2017. https://doi.org/10.1016/j.tcr.2017.10.016.

30. Leblanc MR, Lalonde DH, Thoma A, et al. Is main operating room sterility really necessary in carpal tunnel surgery? A multicenter prospective study of minor procedure room field sterility surgery. Hand (N Y) 2011;6:60–3.

31. Available at: https://walant.surgery/. Accessed March 4, 2018.

Wide-Awake Hand Surgery in Two Centers in China
Experience in Nantong and Tianjin with 12,000 patients

Jin Bo Tang, MD[a],*, Ke Tong Gong, MD[b],
Shu Guo Xing, MD[a], Lu Yi, MD[b], Jian Hua Xu, MD[b]

KEYWORDS

- Anesthesia • Tourniquet • Emergency surgery • Efficiency • Wide awake • Hand surgery
- WALANT • LANT

KEY POINTS

- In China, operations in the upper extremity are commonly performed with brachial plexus block, with a tourniquet applied to the upper arm in awake unsedated patients. Local anesthesia with epinephrine is currently well accepted in China to replace a tourniquet and brachial plexus block for selected groups of patients.
- This article summarizes the cases and application of local anesthesia no tourniquet in 2 large hand surgery centers in Nantong and Tianjin, where more than 12,000 patients were operated on with the new approach over the past 8 years.
- This approach achieves excellent anesthetic and vasoconstrictive effects and is considered the best choice for carpal tunnel release, fixation of digital or metacarpal fractures, primary nerve or tendon repairs, and tendon transfers. The authors have extended this approach to vascularized pedicle flaps and advancement flap transfers.
- In Nantong, surgeons performed a large number of cases of soft tissue benign tumor excision and fracture fixation with this approach. In Tianjin, surgeons applied it to emergency surgeries for hand trauma as well as elective carpal tunnel releases, tendon repair or transfers, and nerve repairs.
- Improvement in efficiency in workflow, decreased wasted time and workload by surgeons, and decreases in patient cost are the major reasons that have led to widespread use of this technique by all surgeons in 2 major hand surgery units. Experience from 2 units with surgery on more than 12,000 patients shows that this approach to surgery is safe, economical, and patient friendly, with no increase in infection rate.

INTRODUCTION

In China, most operations in the upper extremity had been traditionally performed with brachial plexus block in unsedated patients. In these patients, a tourniquet was applied to the upper arm or finger to stop intraoperative bleeding. If the Chinese used a direct translation of "wide-awake hand surgery" to describe this technique, Chinese hand surgeons would wonder why this is new because almost all their patients are traditionally wide awake with no sedation to get their brachial plexus blocks and tourniquet hand surgery.

[a] Department of Hand Surgery, The Hand Surgery Research Center, Affiliated Hospital of Nantong University, 20 West Temple Road, Nantong 226001, Jiangsu, China; [b] Department of Hand Surgery, Tianjin Hospital, 406 Jiefang Nan Road, Hexi District, Tianjin 300211, China
* Corresponding author.
E-mail address: jinbotang@yahoo.com

Hand Clin 35 (2019) 7–12
https://doi.org/10.1016/j.hcl.2018.08.011

What is new about wide-awake hand surgery from a Chinese perspective is that the anesthetic with epinephrine is administered into the operative site locally by the surgeon to achieve both anesthesia and vasoconstriction. Epinephrine eliminates the need for a tourniquet, and this is the momentous change for Chinese surgeons. The tourniquet-free patients have no discomfort and can easily move their digits, hand, and arm actively on the operating table to validate quality of the surgery.[1–6] This technique differs greatly from the traditional practice of simply keeping the patient awake and has gained popularity quickly in China.

Because Chinese patients are traditionally wide awake for hand surgery, most hand surgeons in China agree with the proposal of the lead author (JBT) that the English words, *wide awake*, are not required. Instead, the authors prefer to use the Chinese translation, local anesthesia no tourniquet (LANT), to describe the technique that much of the world has come to know as wide-awake LANT (WALANT).

There are many other countries besides China where patients get hand surgery without sedation and, therefore, have traditionally been wide awake. It may be that LANT is, therefore, a more appropriate term than WALANT for many patients of the world when discussing tourniquet-free hand surgery under local anesthesia.

Chinese hand surgeons recognize 4 basic merits of wide-awake hand surgery:

1. The patient is awake during surgery.
2. No tourniquet is needed.
3. No anesthesiologist is involved.
4. The patient can move the digits, hand, and forearm actively any time during surgery, at the request of the surgeons.

PATIENT DATA IN TWO CENTERS AND SOURCES

In China, the largest number of patients who have had surgery with this approach so far is in Nantong and Tianjin, where more than 12,000 patients have been operated on with this approach.

Hand surgeons in Nantong University started to use this approach in late 2010, with the patients operated on in a minor procedure room in the initial years. The patient data were recorded by operating surgeons, without a trackable hospital-wide system of data collection. The data from the first years, therefore, are not accurate or available. Beginning in 2015, better hospital-wide electronic medical chart and billing systems were introduced

to replace the regional networks in the hospital. This is when the data began to be retrievable with accuracy. The authors estimate that at least 4500 patients had LANT surgery in Nantong over the past 8 years. A total of 935 patients were operated on with this approach in the 1 year before this writing.

Hand surgeons in Tianjin Hospital started the LANT approach of hand surgery in February 2016. Their hospital-wide electronic chart system was already available in 2016. Therefore, the surgeons in Tianjin can track back all their patients. During the first 15 months, they operated on 3107 patients with this approach.[7] The cases are continuously audited. In the 25-month period from February 2016 to March 2018, they operated on a total of 7673 patients with this approach. In the 10 months before this writing, they operated on 4564 patients with the LANT approach.

APPLICATIONS AND UNIQUE TECHNIQUES IN TWO CENTERS

Common procedures that hand surgeons in the 2 centers performed in the wide-awake setting are outlined in **Tables 1** and **2**. Some of this unique experience is described.

Emergency Surgeries with LANT Hand Surgery

In both Nantong and Tianjin, this approach was used extensively in emergency surgical patients. In China, it is common that hand surgeons fix open fractures and perform primary nerve or tendon repairs in an emergency setting, completed within a few hours after patient arrival. Usually 4 to 5 surgeons (2 attending and 2 or 3 trainees) are stationed in the hospital 24 hours a day to operate on these patients immediately after their arrival. This system is efficient. This is different from the system in hospitals in North America, where hand trauma in most patients is seen in emergency rooms where the skin is closed for delayed repair. The merit of the hand surgery system in China is that patients do not need a second procedure after skin closure. LANT surgery lends itself well to the way hand trauma is managed in Nantong and Tianjin because it simplifies even further the trauma management.

LANT internal fixation of open fractures,[7–9] as well as the repair of nerves and tendons,[10–12] decreases the waiting time before surgery and, therefore, recovery time after surgery. In Nantong, approximately 20% of the patients having had LANT hand surgery were for emergency

Table 1 Wide-awake hand surgery data from September 2017 to August 2018 in one theater in Nantong	
Surgical Procedures	Number of Patients
Excision of soft tissue mass	143
Carpal tunnel release	73
Trigger finger release	76
Hand fracture internal fixation/removal	62
Flap transfer	50
Tendon repair	25
Tenolysis	12
Cubital tunnel release	9
Nerve repair	8
Tendon transfer	4
Collateral ligament repair of joints	5
Release of finger joint contracture	4
Local débridement, skin graft, foreign body removal, etc.	149
Total	620

For a patient having multiple procedures in one surgery, only the most complex one is counted.

operations. In Tianjin, about 30% of LANT patients had emergency surgical procedures.

Percentages of the Patients Who Had LANT Hand Surgery

In past 25 months in Tianjin, 26% of the total number of hand surgery patients had LANT hand surgery. This means that 7673 of 29,500 patients who had hand operations in this center had LANT hand surgery. In Nantong, 22% of the surgical patients in the past 12 months had LANT hand surgery. In Tianjin, two-thirds of the patients who had tendon and nerve repairs or transfers in Tianjin had the LANT approach. In Nantong, LANT was used for one-third of these cases.

At Tianjin Hospital, wide-awake hand surgery is now performed every weekday in major operating rooms. Hand surgeons reached a consensus with the department of anesthesiology that local anesthesia is the main form of anesthesia for certain hand disorders, so that an anesthesiologist is not required in those cases. In Nantong, a wide-awake hand surgery theater was built outside of the main operating room on the hand surgery ward, which is entirely managed by the Department of Hand Surgery without anesthesiologists involved.

Percentage of Hand Surgeons Who Accept This Approach

Among hand surgeons in Nantong (14 attending and 14–16 trainees) and in Tianjin (34 attending and trainees), 100% accept and like this approach.

Unique Approaches to LANT Hand Surgery in the Authors' Two Centers

The authors do not wait for 20 minutes to 30 minutes to start surgery

There is level I evidence that it takes 26 minutes for maximal vasoconstriction after lidocaine with epinephrine injection in subcutaneous tissue.[13] The authors have found, however, that waiting only 5 minutes to 15 minutes to start surgery works well. The authors believe that minor bleeding in the surgical field is fine. An entirely bloodless field is not necessary for most procedures; only a field with good visibility is needed. The shorter waiting time for epinephrine vasoconstriction works well. Especially when a patient is injected inside the operating room, the authors do not wait a full 25 minutes to incise the skin. Rather, the first thing done is injecting the local anesthesia. Then, 5 minutes to 10 minutes are spent complete prepping and draping and then proceeding immediately to skin incision (**Fig. 1**). This is especially true for the surgery where the soft tissue over operated structures is thin, such as in extensor tendon surgery (**Figs. 2** and **3**), trigger finger release (**Fig. 4**), and so forth.

A temporary tourniquet for five minutes for patients having open hand trauma

In emergency surgeries for open trauma, some of the authors use a conventional tourniquet in the upper arm for approximately 5 minutes, which can be useful for patients with multiple finger wounds or a large open wound in the hand or forearm. The authors' patients tolerate 5 minutes of tourniquet well.[14,15] The tourniquet use decreases active bleeding at the trauma site and gives the epinephrine 5 minutes to work without washout. Even with only 5 minutes of waiting after injection of epinephrine, the bleeding is much less when the tourniquet is released.

Epinephrine injection can be used in flap harvesting

Surgeons in Nantong apply LANT to flap harvesting[16], which is further detailed in Drs Shu Guo Xing and Jin Bo Tang's article, "Extending Applications of Local Anesthesia Without Tourniquet to Flap Harvest and Transfer in the Hand," in this issue. Surgeons in Tianjin have not used it in flap harvest or transfer. This technique was reported for finger replantation recently.[17]

Table 2
Wide-awake hand surgery data from February 2016 to March 2018 in the hand center in Tianjin

Surgical Procedures	Number of Patients
Emergency surgeries	(5616 patients)
Simple soft tissue repair	1978
Complex soft tissue, arterial exploration/repair	1544
Open fracture reduction and fixation	1380
Tendon and nerve exploration/repair	413
Primary nerve repair	122
Primary flexor tendon repair	92
Primary extensor tendon repair	79
Elective surgeries	(2061 patients)
Soft tissue tumor excision: hand	389
Upper and forearm	120
Open reduction and internal fixation	340
Internal fixation removal	320
Carpal tunnel release	370[a]
Cubital tunnel release	110
Tendon repair or tenolysis	52
Tendon transfer	25
Treatment of closed tendon ruptures	45[b]
Trigger fingers and mallet fingers	290
Total	7673

[a] One patient had ulnar nerve release at Guyon canal.
[b] Fifteen patients had flexor pollicis longus tendon ruptures due to distal radius fracture, 12 flexor tendon ruptures due to steroid injection or percutaneous trigger finger release, 8 tendon ruptures due to rheumatoid arthritis of the hand, and 8 ruptures of flexor digitorum profundus tendons at the insertion.

Brachial plexus anesthesia with epinephrine and no tourniquet

The surgeons in Tianjin like a hybrid of a brachial plexus block and injection of epinephrine for surgery in the elbow and upper arm, which they call "brachial plexus anesthesia epinephrine no tourniquet." They like it for cubital tunnel release. This hybrid gives a wide anesthesia field. In addition, epinephrine permits early removal of the tourniquet, which allows more space for surgery. In Nantong, hand surgeons inject local anesthesia and

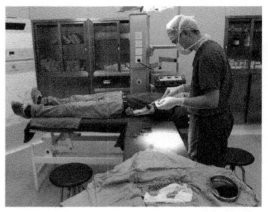

Fig. 1. A typical operative setting in Nantong. The local anesthestic is injected on the operating table. The surgeon proceeds to sterilization and draping, which take approximately 5 to 10 minutes. Then the surgeon proceeds to the surgical procedure without additional waiting time for most patients.

epinephrine for cubital tunnel release without a brachial plexus block and without a tourniquet.

Supplementary anesthesia to deeper tissues is needed during some procedures

In performing open reduction and internal fixation of the metacarpus or phalanges, or removing tumors from these bones, an additional 10 mL to 20 mL of 1% lidocaine is infused onto the periosteum and the bone cavity to reduce pain or discomfort. If local anesthetic is only administered to the skin and subcutaneous tissue, sometimes it does not efficiently anesthetize the bone. In addition, median, ulnar, and digital nerve blocks can be helpful to ensure that patients remain pain-free. The larger the nerve, however, the longer it takes for nerve blocks to work. Tumescent

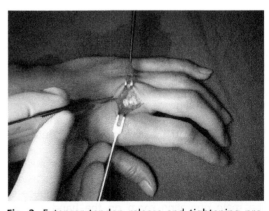

Fig. 2. Extensor tendon release and tightening procedure, 10 minutes after injection. This quick, good surgical field with much reduced blood provides a sufficiently clean field for surgery.

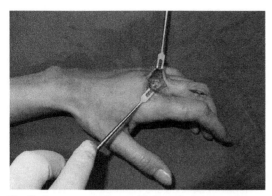

Fig. 3. Extensor tendon and joint release surgeries are suitable for a short waiting time after injection of local anesthetics with epinephrine.

anesthesia works quickly by anesthetizing all the small nerves in the operated area.

Converting the patient experience of surgery to a movie theater experience

In Nantong, the patient waiting area contains a station for patients to pick up popular movies or music stored in hard drives or iPads. Inside the operating room, patients can enjoy watching movies with earphones during their surgery. They are placed in a reclining position, extending their hand for the surgeons to operate on. This setting entirely transforms the patient's potentially psychologically stressful surgery into a movie theater experience. Many patients have told surgeons that they had an unexpectedly pleasant experience in the wide-awake hand surgery theater. They feel thankful to the surgeons and nurses.

Safety of This Procedure in Two Centers

In both centers, there has not been an increase in infection rates after surgery compared with the

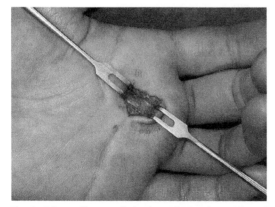

Fig. 4. Trigger finger release in wide-awake setting of the same patient shown in **Fig. 3**.

previous conventional approach. In Nantong, phentolamine is used occasionally after surgery to negate the fear of white digits in some patients. None of the patients suffered epinephrine-induced tissue necrosis or loss. In Tianjin, phentolamine was not used in any of the 7673 patients and the surgeons found no epinephrine injection–related tissue necrosis in their patients.

HOW TO INCREASE THE POPULARITY OF LANT
Surgeons' Willingness is a Key

A positive attitude of the surgeons, especially senior surgeons, and their willingness to use the LANT technique are key to facilitate permitting more patients to benefit from its advantages. Once 1 or 2 surgeons in a team start to use this approach, the others quickly see its benefits and will follow. Dr Ke Tong Gong, chair of the hand surgery service in Tianjin Hospital, said, "At the beginning, it was me who wanted the other surgeons to do it. After just a few months, it was they who wanted to use it, to modify it, to teach other how to do it better, and to spread the message." He further added, "All in the department are doing LANT and they all like it!" In Nantong, all the hand surgeons use it because they see the efficiency. In both units, the authors believe that the chairpersons' encouragement is an important driving force.

Conferences, symposiums, and courses

Over the past 4 years, congresses and forums for hand surgeons organized by the lead author (JBT) have regularly included courses or symposiums on wide-awake hand surgery. More than 600 hand surgeons in China have attended these courses or symposiums. The attendees have become the major driving force in increasing the popularity of this technique in China. This has been boosted by the Chinese version of the book, *Wide Awake Hand Surgery*[18], which was published in 2017. This Chinese publication is a combination of some of Dr Lalonde's original book and video contents plus the addition of the experience gained in China.

FUTURE PERSPECTIVES

In China, hand surgeons are very interested in the use of epinephrine injection to replace the tourniquet. Local anesthesia is a way of saving of medical resources and costs.[19] These are great benefits. Because of the diverse landscape of the country, surgeons working in more inland areas have not yet begun to use this approach. The authors expect that the popularity of this technique will increase in those areas over time. Chinese hand surgeons have less resistance to this technique than seen in some other countries. Chinese patients are willing to undergo surgeries under local anesthesia. The administrative system also welcomes the innovative approach, because it benefits the hospital, surgeons, and patients through improved efficiency in treatment, better distribution of resources, and savings in materials and cost. The authors expect further popularization in the next few years.

SUMMARY

Chinese hand surgeons have quickly adopted the LANT approach to hand surgery. Two units in China have used it in more than 120,000 patients over the past 8 years. The authors have found it safe in patients and are now using this approach for 20% to 30% of all hand surgery patients. The 2 units have added the new dimensions of flap surgery, a shorter waiting time after injection, temporary tourniquet use at the start of the surgery, and hybrid brachial plexus block plus epinephrine injection. In the 2 units, all the hand surgeons use this approach in emergency and elective operations. The authors have found it a useful way to reduce patients' medical costs as well as surgeon workload. LANT has increased work efficiency in the authors' hand surgery centers.

REFERENCES

1. Lalonde DH, Wong A. Dosage of local anesthesia in wide awake hand surgery. J Hand Surg Am 2013;38: 2025–8.
2. Lalonde DH. Wide-awake flexor tendon repair. Plast Reconstr Surg 2009;123:623–5.
3. Lalonde D, Higgins A. Wide awake flexor tendon repair in the finger. Plast Reconstr Surg Glob Open 2016;4:e797.
4. Lalonde DH. Conceptual origins, current practice, and views of wide awake hand surgery. J Hand Surg Eur Vol 2017;42:886–95.
5. Lalonde D. Minimally invasive anesthesia in wide awake hand surgery. Hand Clin 2014;30:1–6.
6. Gong KT, Xing SG. How to establish and standardize wide-awake hand surgery: experience from China. J Hand Surg Eur Vol 2017;42:868–70.
7. Xing SG, Tang JB. Surgical treatment, hardware removal, and the wide-awake approach for metacarpal fractures. Clin Plast Surg 2014;41:463–80.
8. Tang JB, Gong KT, Zhu L, et al. Performing hand surgery under local anesthesia without a tourniquet in china. Hand Clin 2017;33:415–24.
9. Liodaki E, Xing SG, Mailaender P, et al. Management of difficult intra-articular fractures or fracture dislocations of the proximal interphalangeal joint. J Hand Surg Eur Vol 2015;40:16–23.
10. Zhou X, Qing J, Chen J. Outcomes of the 6-strand M-Tang repair for zone 2 primary flexor tendon repair in 54 fingers. J Hand Surg Eur Vol 2017;42: 462–8.
11. Pan ZJ, Qin J, Zhou X, et al. Robust thumb flexor tendon repairs with a six-strand M-Tang method, pulley venting, and early active motion. J Hand Surg Eur Vol 2017;42:909–14.
12. Tang JB. Wide-awake primary flexor tendon repair, tenolysis and tendon transfer. Clin Orthop Surg 2015;7:275–81.
13. McKee DE, Lalonde DH, Thoma A, et al. Optimal time delay between epinephrine injection and incision to minimize bleeding. Plast Reconstr Surg 2013;131:811.
14. Xing SG, Mao T. The use of local anaesthesia with epinephrine in the harvest and transfer of an extended Segmuller flap in the fingers. J Hand Surg Eur Vol 2018;43:783–4.
15. Iqbal HJ, Doorgakant A, Rehmatullah NNT, et al. Pain and outcomes of carpal tunnel release under local anaesthetic with or without a tourniquet: a randomized controlled trial. J Hand Surg Eur Vol 2018; 43:808–12.
16. Xing SG, Mao T. Temporary tourniquet use after epinephrine injection to expedite wide awake emergency hand surgeries. J Hand Surg Eur Vol 2018;43: 888–9.
17. Wong J, Lin CH, Chang NJ, et al. Digital revascularization and replantation using the wide-awake hand surgery technique. J Hand Surg Eur Vol 2017;42: 621–5.
18. Tang JB. Wide awake hand surgery. Shanghai (China): Shanghai Scientific & Technical Publishers; 2017.
19. Rhee PC, Fischer MM, Rhee LS, et al. Cost savings and patient experiences of a clinic-Based, wide-awake hand surgery program at a military medical center: a critical analysis of the first 100 procedures. J Hand Surg Am 2017;42:e139–47.

The Current and Possible Future Role of Wide-Awake Local Anesthesia No Tourniquet Hand Surgery in Military Health Care Delivery

Peter Charles Rhee, DO, MS

KEYWORDS

- Wide-awake hand surgery • WALANT • Military health care • Echelon of care
- Damage control orthopedic • Humanitarian hand surgery

KEY POINTS

- The ability to perform hand surgery without general or sedating anesthesia conserves limited anesthetic resources and allows patients to maintain situational awareness perioperatively.
- WALANT hand surgery for isolated hand trauma in areas of combat may even enable troops to remain in a deployed setting, with a brief period of restricted duties, to maintain a healthy fight force in theater.
- For humanitarian care to local nationals whose medical history is often unknown, WALANT hand surgery obviates preoperative medical clearance.
- The tremendous cost-savings and surgical efficiency associated with WALANT hand surgery can enhance the access to hand surgery care for soldiers and veterans within the military health care system.
- Clinic-based hand surgery benefits patients by reducing their costs, increasing their convenience, enhancing access to care, and optimizing safety with the elimination of sedation.

INTRODUCTION

The concept of wide-awake local anesthesia no tourniquet (WALANT) hand surgery is well aligned with the surgical goal of initiating early range of motion to more rapidly restore function.[1,2] In addition to the benefits of incurring less cost for the military health care system (MHS) with performing hand surgery under WALANT in the clinic versus the main operating room, the ability to perform procedures with no preoperative testing or perioperative sedation can be extremely beneficial to the military population and their beneficiaries.[3,4] Wide-awake hand surgery has tremendous applicability in military medicine and can be used in many operational settings.[3] This article discusses the current and possible role of wide-awake hand surgery in military health care delivery.

ARENAS OF MILITARY HAND SURGERY

In military medicine, hand surgery can be delivered in a variety of settings with their own unique challenges. In the domestic setting, active duty soldiers and veterans are entitled to hand surgery through the MHS and represent the largest burden of care in terms of resource expenditure

Disclosure Statement: None of the authors have disclosures to declare.
Division of Hand Surgery, Department of Orthopedic Surgery, Mayo Clinic, 200 First Street Southwest, Rochester, MN 55905, USA
E-mail address: rhee.peter@mayo.edu

Hand Clin 35 (2019) 13–19
https://doi.org/10.1016/j.hcl.2018.08.008

and limiting the access to care.[3] In the operational setting, military medical efforts are aimed at supporting soldiers in areas of combat or toward providing humanitarian care to local nationals (LNs) in foreign countries for many diplomatic reasons. In most combat injuries, performing definitive hand surgery is often inhibited by the medical instability of the patient, the need to treat more severe injuries in polytrauma patients, and the demand to ration surgical supplies for other emergent procedures. Similarly, in humanitarian efforts, the underlying medical comorbidities of LNs are often unknown or poorly managed, which can create difficulties with administering general or intravenous (IV) sedation anesthesia. Wide-awake hand surgery can be applied in all of these unique care settings in military medicine.

Combat Zones

Various echelons of medical care have been developed to provide sequential and effective treatment to soldiers injured in areas of combat.[5] Each echelon of care is designed with increasing medical capabilities to adequately treat complex injuries. The early focus is on saving life, limb, and eyesight while providing only the essentials of care until the patient is transferred to a higher echelon of medical support.[5] As a patient transfers and progresses through the various echelons, every effort is made to avoid interventions that may confound the next stage of treatment.[5] The echelons or levels of medical care for the US military and most foreign militaries are outlined in **Table 1**.

Injuries sustained in combat zones can be classified as battle injuries (BIs) or nonbattle injuries (NBIs), with the latter causing a considerable loss of able-bodied service members from the operational theater.[6] Hauret and colleagues[6] evaluated the frequency and causes of NBIs in US Army soldiers that required medical air evacuation from Operation Iraqi Freedom (OIF, Iraq) and Operation Enduring Freedom (OEF, Afghanistan) from 2001 until 2006. Of the 27,563 air evacuations from OIF, 34.6% (9530 cases) were from NBIs versus 18% (4968 cases) from BIs. Similarly, of the 4165 air evacuations from OEF, 36.4% (1515 cases) were NBIs versus 10.4% (433 cases) from BIs. The top 3 causes for NBIs in Iraq and Afghanistan were as follows:

1. Sports and physical training
2. Falls/jumps
3. Motor vehicle–related incidents.[6]

Most NBIs sustained in combat zones involves the upper extremity.[6,7] During OIF and OEF,

NBIs to the wrist, hand, or fingers accounted for 15.3% (770 of 5035) and 16.6% (136 of 817) of the total number of causes for air evacuations of US Army soldiers out of both operational theaters.[6] The most common cause for NBIs was fractures in Iraq (18.9%) and Afghanistan (18.8%). Similarly, of the 491 upper extremity injuries in French military soldiers treated at a level 3 combat support hospital (Kabul International Airport) from 2009 until 2013, 50.3% (n = 247) of soldiers had sustained an NBI that was predominantly work related (46%, n = 114).[7] Of the 148 NBIs to the hand, the type of injuries consisted of soft tissue injuries (n = 71), open fractures (n = 33), closed fractures (n = 22), traumatic amputations (n = 13), and burns (n = 9). These studies illustrate the high propensity of non-battle-related fractures in the hand that often necessitates air evacuations and repatriation of soldiers out of combat.

Closed metacarpal fractures are common NBIs sustained by service members in the military that can result in considerable time away from duties.[8] During a 10-month period, Greer[9] observed 76 metacarpal fractures in 64 US military soldiers assigned to an installation in South Korea. In that study, 63% of fractures (n = 48) occurred to the fifth metacarpal, and the cause of injury was commonly due to anger or an altercation (45%, n = 29) and physical training (22%, n = 14). Dichiera and colleagues[8] noted 367 metacarpal fractures in US Army soldiers, of which 76% (n = 277) affected the fifth metacarpal and were most commonly self-inflicted by punching an object. Greer[9] estimated that each metacarpal fracture accounted for approximately 98 hours of time lost at work, 360 hours of reduced job performance, and 909 hours (38 days) of restricted duties from the US military.[8,9]

Although definitive surgical treatment of metacarpal and phalangeal fractures is typically not the current goal in early echelons of care, performing these procedures in level 2 and 3 medical facilities can maintain a healthy fighting force in the operational theater. Penn-Barnwell and colleagues[10] reported on 153 UK soldiers with isolated hand injuries, consisting of closed (n = 67) and open (16) fractures, while deployed to Iraq or Afghanistan over a 6-year period.[10] All patients with hand fractures required repatriation to the United Kingdom to have their definitive fracture management at a level 5 medical facility, thus removing 83 soldiers from their deployed locations.[10] However, many of those soldiers underwent initial temporizing care (surgical debridement, closed reduction, splint

Table 1
United States military echelons of medical care

Level of Care	Location	Type of Medical Care/ Facilities	Medical Roles/Capabilities
1	• Battlefield	• Self-care • First responders • Battalion aid stations • Shock trauma platoons	• Typically performed by the wounded or their immediate combat colleague • Lifesaving techniques (application of tourniquets, pressure dressings, hemostatic agents) • Prevent the "lethal triad" of hypothermia, coagulopathy, and hypotension • Basic and advanced cardiopulmonary resuscitation
2	• Near the zone of combat	• Forward surgical units • Forward resuscitative surgical systems	• Resuscitative, life-saving procedures (laparotomy, tracheostomy, and so forth) • Limb-saving procedures (irrigation, debridement, amputation, vascular shunting, external fixation)

3	• Region of combat
	• In theater
		• Field hospital
		• Combat support hospital
		• Evacuation hospital
			• Stabilize soldiers for rapid evacuation
			• Soldiers:
			  ○ Emergent and urgent procedures before transportation (irrigation, debridement, amputation, definitive vessel repair/reconstruction, external fixation)
			  ○ Definitive care for minor injuries[a]
			• LNs:
			  ○ Definitive surgical care for all injuries

4	• Overseas • Out of theater	• Medical treatment facility	• Definitive surgical care[a] • Ongoing temporizing procedures for staged definitive surgical care
5	• Continental United States • Out of theater	• Large medical center	• Definitive surgical care and rehabilitation

[a] Based on the capabilities of the surgical personnel present, resources available, and the operational tempo of the medical facility at a given time.

immobilization) by an orthopedic surgeon at a forward surgical unit (level 2) where the opportunity to perform definitive care was lost.

Wide-awake hand surgery can facilitate the delivery of hand fracture care in the austere environment to keep soldiers in the operational theater. The unique benefit of performing closed reduction, phalangeal and metacarpal fractures fixation under WALANT is the ability to confirm fracture stability intraoperatively with active motion under fluoroscopy, that can permit early protected movement resulting in an expedited recovery and return to full active duties.[2,11] Poggetti and colleagues[12] reported on 25 metacarpals stabilized with intramedullary headless compression screw fixation under WALANT that resulted in radiographic union for all cases at a mean of 4.4 weeks

after starting early active motion with only buddy strapping to the adjacent digit immediately postoperatively. Practically, a service member with a closed hand fracture can undergo WALANT hand surgery, recover "behind the wire" out of combat, remain in the operational theater performing restricted duties, with an anticipated return to full duties in a shorter timeframe then to select, train, and deploy a replacement for the injured soldier.

In early echelons of care, WALANT hand surgery may be beneficial to minimize the use of opioids medications postoperatively and to eliminate the development of altered mental status after IV sedation or general anesthesia. Ramirez and colleagues[13] reported that 31% of active duty service members admitted to opioid misuse with a higher risk in those who suffer from posttraumatic stress disorder from a recent deployment. Therefore, decreasing perioperative anxiety and pain may reduce the need for opioid use postoperatively. Davison and colleagues[14] noted that patients undergoing carpal tunnel release (CTR) had significantly less mean perioperatively anxiety (0 = no anxiety and 10 = worst anxiety) when the procedure was performed under WALANT compared with IV sedation (2.3 vs 3.4, $P = .007$). Gunasagaran and colleagues[15] observed less mean pain on the visual analogue score (VAS) with CTR (n = 8), A1 pulley release (APR, n = 30), and ganglion cyst excision (n = 2) performed under WALANT (VAS = 2.33) compared with local anesthesia and tourniquet use (VAS = 4.72, $P<.05$). Miller and colleagues[16] reported that patients who underwent wide-awake open CTR or APR were less likely to take opioids (49% vs 62%, $P = .01$) and use them for less days (mean of 1.61 vs 1.83 days, $P = .03$) compared with patients who had the same procedures performed under IV sedation. Less risk of opioid misuse, decreased periprocedural anxiety, and no postoperative altered mental status from systemic anesthesia support the use of wide-awake surgery in combat zones to optimize the emotional health of the injured soldier.

Wide-awake hand surgery can obviate damage control surgery in isolated hand trauma at a level 2 or 3 medical facility. The term damage control orthopedic (DCO) surgery is directed at the initial phase of treatment that focuses on controlling hemorrhage, minimizing wound contamination, and temporarily stabilizing fractures in polytrauma patients with hemodynamic instability.[17] In combat hand trauma, the main objectives of DCO are to prevent infection and to perform a detailed exploration to prepare for staged secondary repair at a high echelon of care.[18] Definitive hand surgery should not be performed in the austere environment for severely traumatized extremities with extensive vascular, bone, or soft tissue injuries.[17] However, for many nonemergent hand NBIs without these associated injuries, such as closed hand fractures and finger lacerations with tendon involvement, transfer to a level 4 or 5 medical facility for definitive treatment can be delayed for 3 to 4 days due to operational constraints and can result in suboptimal surgical outcomes.[10,19] Similarly, with limited personnel in forward surgical units and combat support hospitals, anesthesia providers may be unavailable to perform IV sedation or general anesthesia for hand surgery procedures. This particular scenario presents an opportunity to perform wide-awake hand fracture care and tendon repairs with minimal constraints on ancillary support.[1,2]

In appropriate situations, emergent replantation and revascularization in the hand can be performed in the austere setting.[19] Most digit amputations in combat zones are the result of crush or blast mechanisms and are not indicated for replantation. Otherwise, sharp digit amputations and lacerations resulting in critical ischemia are rare in combat. Brininger and colleagues[20] noted that digit amputations accounted for less than 0.2% of the upper extremity injuries sustained by the US military and are often work related. However, in soldiers who have sustained injuries that require microsurgical reconstruction, sequential patient transfer from a level 2 to a level 4 facility may take many hours to days, thus eliminating any possibility for digit salvage. Based on the experiences of a French Forward Surgical Unit (level 2), Mathieu and colleagues[19] proposed a treatment algorithm advocating replantation or revascularization in the combat zone for midpalmar or proximal hand level complete amputations or for dysvascular partial amputations. For thumb or multiple digit amputations, they recommended immediate transfer to a level 4 or 5 facility and delayed transfer for single finger amputations.

With the proper surgical assets and instruments, wide-awake hand surgery can enable the execution of digit replantation or revascularization in early echelons of care. In level 2 medical facilities, the supply of IV and inhaled anesthetic medications is limited and must be reserved for life-threatening injuries and other emergent procedures that warrant general anesthesia or IV sedation. Performing microsurgery on the ischemic or amputated digit under WALANT preserves those valuable resources. Mathieu and colleagues[19] described the case of successful replantation of a distal phalanx amputation under local anesthesia with the use of microsurgical instruments and ×3.5 magnification loupes on the flight deck of an French aircraft carrier (level 2). Wong and colleagues[21] reported on 5 cases of revascularization and 8 replantations under WALANT, consisting of 2% lidocaine with 1:100,000 adrenaline injected into the digit. All digits survived without the need for reoperation, allowing the authors to conclude that wide-awake digit revascularization and replantation is safe and should be considered for patients who are at risk for medical complications with general anesthesia, if immediate anesthetic support is unavailable, or if the patient declines general or regional anesthesia.

Humanitarian Missions

The US military often provides medical care to LNs in areas of combat or to citizens in developing foreign countries that are underserved. Providing humanitarian medical care to LNs is not permitted in forward surgical units or combat support hospitals, level 2 and 3. However, if an LN sustains injuries as collateral damage from military efforts, then they are often treated by military medical providers. In this situation, the host country may not have a medical facility with a higher level of care that is accessible for the LN; therefore, definitive surgical treatment can be delivered to the patient. Another situation where the US military can provide medical care to LNs is through medical readiness training exercises (MEDRETE). The MEDRETEs are an opportunity for medical teams to train and practice medicine in challenging and austere environments, treat medical conditions not common encountered in the US population, develop stronger relationship with the host country, and provide medical care to an underserved native population.[22] In fiscal year 2009, the US Army conducted 89 MEDRETEs in 18 countries, treating approximately 235,000 LNs.[22]

Transportation and acquisition of inhaled anesthetic medications in remote areas can be difficult; thus, the delivery of general or IV sedation anesthesia remains a limiting factor in the number of procedures that can be performed. Doman and colleagues[22] noted that despite meticulous predeployment planning, a US Army hand surgery MEDRETE arrived at their mission site, yet all preoperative antibiotics and sedation medications (Propofol) did not arrive. However, they were able to perform 58 hand surgical cases under local anesthesia and judicious use of alternative sedatives that were hand carried with the mission team. Nugent and colleagues[23] also stressed the importance of having providers on the surgical team for humanitarian missions who are comfortable with both delivering anesthetic blocks and performing surgery with no or minimal sedation to circumvent the need for potentially limited anesthetic agents that should be rationed. These experiences illustrate the benefit of WALANT hand surgery in maximizing the number of cases that can be performed in host countries due to conservation of anesthetic resources.

Wide-awake hand surgery can address some of the perioperative anesthetic challenges encountered in the care of LNs in foreign countries. Because of substandard or often unavailable preventative medical care in developing and war torn countries, LNs can have multiple comorbidities that are undiagnosed and undertreated, which can place them at risk for anesthetic complications. Oftentimes, LNs are unable to provide a medical history, and preoperative medical tests cannot be readily performed (electrocardiogram, complete blood count, basic metabolic panel, chest radiograph, and cardiac stress tests). Therefore, general or IV sedation must be delivered cautiously with expectant management with prolonged postanesthesia monitoring. A benefit of WALANT hand surgery in this scenario is the ability to perform safe and effective hand surgery without preoperative medical clearance. In addition, without the administration of sedating medications, patients can received clear postoperative rehabilitative plans through an interpreter perioperatively, and the anxiety of "falling asleep" among strangers is curtailed. Furthermore, LNs often present for surgery without a companion, thus without the administration of sedatives, patients can safely discharge on their own without the aid of a family member or friend. Last, the expedient postoperative recovery relieves the burden of monitoring by anesthesia providers and can facilitate faster patient turnover from the post-anesthetic care unit.

Military Medical Treatment Facilities in the Continental United States

In recent years, there has been limited access to hand surgery care for veterans, active duty soldiers, and their dependents.[3] In the CONUS (Continental United States), hand surgery for military beneficiaries is delivered at military treatment facilities (MTFs) that are sparsely situated throughout the country. Because of a limited number of hand surgeons in the US military and shortage in operating room availability at MTFs, patients are often deferred to civilian hand surgeons who are compensated through a military health care plan (TRICARE) that is comparable to Medicare and Medicaid. With an operating cost of $52.7 billion, or 13% of the Department of Defense budget, to cover 10 million beneficiaries, the financial burden of deferring patients "out of networks" places considerable fiscal strains on the MHS.[3,24,25] However, wide-awake hand surgery may facilitate more surgical cases in a given period of time thus improving access to hand surgery for beneficiaries at an MTF. Leblanc and colleagues[4] reported the ability to perform 9 CTRs compared with 4 CTRs under WALANT in an ambulatory setting versus in the operating room during a 3-hour surgical block, respectively. Similarly, Rhee and colleagues[3] noted that 2 to 3 elective soft tissue cases (CTR, AOR, and de Quervain release) could be performed in an hour with WALANT in a clinic-based setting in an MTF.

Performing WALANT hand surgery in an MTF can result in considerable cost savings for the US MHS.[3] A prospective cohort study performed at a single military medical center noted nearly 85% and 70% cost savings by performing CTR and APR, respectively, in the clinic setting under wide-awake technique compared with the main operating room.[3] By performing CTR, APR, and de Quervain releases in the clinic instead of the main operating room during the 21-month study period, a single MTF was able to save $393,100.[3] Similarly, Codding and colleagues[26] noted that APR performed under wide-awake technique versus monitored anesthetic care in the operating room resulted in significantly less time in the recovery room with WALANT, which amounted to less indirect costs and a minimum cost savings of $105 from direct excess anesthesia charges.

SUMMARY

Wide-awake hand surgery has tremendous applicability and benefits in the various health care settings that are unique to military medicine. In the operational theater, WALANT is advantageous given the ability to perform hand surgery worldwide unencumbered by operating room or anesthesia availability. The lack of perioperative sedation while performing WALANT hand surgery allows soldiers to stay focused and alert postoperatively. When providing hand surgery to LNs, whose medical history is often unknown, wide-awake hand surgery may minimize the risk of anesthesia-related medical complications. Last, the efficiency in surgical turnover associated with WALANT permits enhanced access to hand surgery care for military health care beneficiaries in the CONUS while saving considerable costs for the MHS. The future role of WALANT in military medicine is truly in the hands of military hand surgeons to innovate and advance the current utilization of wide-awake hand surgery to ultimately improve outcomes for soldiers and veterans.

REFERENCES

1. Lalonde DH, Martin AL. Wide-awake flexor tendon repair and early tendon mobilization in zones 1 and 2. Hand Clin 2013;29:207–13.
2. Gregory S, Lalonde DH, Fung Leung LT. Minimally invasive finger fracture management: wide-awake closed reduction, K-wire fixation, and early protected movement. Hand Clin 2014;30:7–15.
3. Rhee PC, Fischer MM, Rhee LS, et al. Cost savings and patient experiences of a clinic-based, wide-awake hand surgery program at a military medical center: a critical analysis of the first 100 procedures. J Hand Surg Am 2017;42:e139–47.
4. Leblanc MR, Lalonde J, Lalonde DH. A detailed cost and efficiency analysis of performing carpal tunnel surgery in the main operating room versus the ambulatory setting in Canada. Hand (N Y) 2007;2: 173–8.
5. Hofmeister EP, Mazurek M, Ingari J. Injuries sustained to the upper extremity due to modern warfare and the evolution of care. J Hand Surg Am 2007;32: 1141–7.
6. Hauret KG, Taylor BJ, Clemmons NS, et al. Frequency and causes of nonbattle injuries air evacuated from operations iraqi freedom and enduring freedom, u.s. Army, 2001-2006. Am J Prev Med 2010;38(1 Suppl):S94–107.
7. Mathieu L, Bertani A, Gaillard C, et al. Wartime upper extremity injuries: experience from the Kabul International Airport combat support hospital. Chir Main 2014;33:183–8.
8. Dichiera R, Dunn J, Bader J, et al. Characterization of metacarpal fractures in a military population. Mil Med 2016;181:931–4.
9. Greer MA. Incidence of metacarpal fractures in U.S. soldiers stationed in South Korea. J Hand Ther 2008; 21:137–41.
10. Penn-Barwell JG, Bennett PM, Powers D, et al. Isolated hand injuries on operational deployment: an examination of epidemiology and treatment strategy. Mil Med 2011;176:1404–7.
11. Xing SG, Tang JB. Surgical treatment, hardware removal, and the wide-awake approach for metacarpal fractures. Clin Plast Surg 2014;41:463–80.
12. Poggetti A, Nucci AM, Giesen T, et al. Percutaneous intramedullary headless screw fixation and wide-awake anesthesia to treat metacarpal fractures: early results in 25 patients. J Hand Microsurg 2018;10:16–21.
13. Ramirez S, Bebarta VS, Varney SM, et al. Misuse of prescribed pain medication in a military population-a self-reported survey to assess a correlation with age, deployment, combat illnesses, or injury? Am J Ther 2017;24:e150–6.
14. Davison PG, Cobb T, Lalonde DH. The patient's perspective on carpal tunnel surgery related to the type of anesthesia: a prospective cohort study. Hand (N Y) 2013;8:47–53.
15. Gunasagaran J, Sean ES, Shivdas S, et al. Perceived comfort during minor hand surgeries with wide awake local anaesthesia no tourniquet (WALANT) versus local anaesthesia (LA)/tourniquet. J Orthop Surg (Hong Kong) 2017;25. 2309499017739499.
16. Miller A, Kim N, Ilyas AM. Prospective evaluation of opioid consumption following hand surgery performed wide awake versus with sedation. Hand (N Y) 2017;12:606–9.
17. Choufani C, Barbier O, Grosset A, et al. Initial management of complex hand injuries in military or austere environments: how to defer and prepare for definitive repair? Int Orthop 2017;41: 1771–5.

18. Jabaley ME, Peterson HD. Early treatment of war wounds of the hand and forearm in Vietnam. Ann Surg 1973;177:167–73.
19. Mathieu L, Levadoux M, Landevoisin ES, et al. Digital replantation in forward surgical units: a cases study. SICOT J 2018;4:9.
20. Brininger TL, Antczak A, Breland HL. Upper extremity injuries in the U.S. military during peacetime years and wartime years. J Hand Ther 2008;21:115–22.
21. Wong J, Lin CH, Chang NJ, et al. Digital revascularization and replantation using the wide-awake hand surgery technique. J Hanfd Surg Eur Vol 2017;42:621–5.
22. Doman DM, Blair JA, Napierala MA, et al. Do plans and execution agree in a humanitarian medical mission? J Surg Orthop Adv 2011;20:67–73.
23. Nugent AG, Panthaki Z, Thaller S. The planning and execution of surgical hand mission trips in developing countries. J Craniofac Surg 2015;26:1055–7.
24. Stinner DJ, Sathiyakumar V, Ficke JR. The military health care system: providing quality care at a low per capita cost. J Orthop Trauma 2014;28(Suppl 10):S11–3.
25. Beauvais B, Wells R, Vasey J, et al. Does money really matter? The effects of fiscal margin on quality of care in military treatment facilities. Hosp Top 2007;85:2–15.
26. Codding JL, Bhat SB, Ilyas AM. An Economic analysis of mac versus walant: a trigger finger release surgery case Study. Hand (N Y) 2017;12:348–51.

The Canadian Model for Instituting Wide-Awake Hand Surgery in Our Hospitals

Margie Wheelock, MD, FRCSC[a],*, Christian Petropolis, MD, FRCSC[b],
Donald H. Lalonde, MSc, DSc, MD, FRCSC[c]

KEYWORDS

- Hand surgery • Local anesthesia • Canada • Treatment costs • WALANT • Field sterility
- Wide awake • No tourniquet

KEY POINTS

- Hand surgery in Canada has evolved over the past 50 years with a progression toward clinic-based wide-awake tourniquet-free hand surgery at many centers.
- Benefits of clinic-based surgery include expedited patient care, reduced health system costs, and offloading of other health system resources, such as in-patient beds and main operating room time.
- Eliminating the sedation, the tourniquet, and surgery at night is safer for patients.
- Clinic-based hand surgery benefits the surgeon by providing a readily available setting for daytime management of both traumatic and elective hand cases.
- Clinic-based hand surgery benefits patients by reducing their costs, and increasing their convenience, access of care, and safety with the elimination of sedation.

INTRODUCTION AND HISTORICAL PERSPECTIVE

Wide-awake hand surgery is based on the premise that epinephrine vasoconstriction eliminates the need for the tourniquet. The myth that epinephrine causes finger necrosis is now clearly dispelled.[1–5] However, many Canadians never believed it in the first place. They therefore used epinephrine with lidocaine in the finger, which enabled them to perform hand surgery without a tourniquet more than 50 years ago.

When Dr Lalonde was a medical student at Queen's University in Kingston, Canada, from 1975 to 1979, the plastic surgeon Dr Patrick Shoemaker, used lidocaine and epinephrine in the finger to regularly perform wide-awake flexor tendon repair and other hand surgery procedures with field sterility in the emergency department. He was the one who convinced Dr Lalonde that epinephrine in the finger is clinically safe.

Dr Bob MacFarlane of London, Canada, was a past president of the American Society for Surgery of the Hand. He was famous for his research in

Disclosure Statement: None of the authors have disclosures to declare. Dr D. Lalonde has edited the *Wide Awake Hand Surgery* book published by Thieme, but all profits go to the Lean and Green effort of the American Association for Hand Surgery dedicated to decrease unnecessary cost and garbage production in hand surgery.
[a] Department of Plastic and Reconstructive Surgery, Dalhousie University, IWK Health Centre, 5850/5980 University Avenue, PO Box 9700, Halifax, Nova Scotia B3K6R8, Canada; [b] Department of Plastic and Reconstructive Surgery, University of Manitoba, Winnipeg Health Sciences Centre, RR445, 800 Sherbrook Street, Winnipeg, Manitoba R3A1R9, Canada; [c] Department of Plastic and Reconstructive Surgery, Dalhousie University, Suite C204, 600 Main Street, Saint John, New Brunswick E2K1J5, Canada
* Corresponding author.
E-mail address: margaret.wheelock@iwk.nshealth.ca

Hand Clin 35 (2019) 21–27
https://doi.org/10.1016/j.hcl.2018.08.001
0749-0712/19/© 2018 Elsevier Inc. All rights reserved.

Dupuytren surgery. He regularly performed wide-awake Dupuytren fasciectomy with lidocaine and epinephrine in the finger his whole career.

OTTAWA

Dr John Fielding, the first plastic surgeon in Canada's capital Ottawa (population 1.3 million), pioneered the use of wide-awake hand surgery with epinephrine hemostasis in the finger in that city beginning in the 1960s. He used lidocaine and epinephrine to perform most hand and finger trauma surgery, such as tendon repair and fracture K wiring, without a tourniquet outside of the main operating room with field sterility in minor procedure rooms and in the emergency departments. His infection rates were always very acceptable. Most of the hand surgeons in Ottawa followed his lead because of the simplicity and the readily available space to do the surgery in the emergency departments. They eliminated the need to admit patients with hand trauma to a bed in the hospital where the patients would need to line up for days to get evening or night operating time in the main operating room. As a result, there is now a whole generation of Ottawa hand surgeons who have almost never taken minor hand surgery to the main operating room.

With the efforts of Drs Murray Allen and Danny Peters, Ottawa built a new wide-awake surgery center adjacent to the emergency department at the Civic Campus of the Ottawa Hospital in 2014. This center has low-power X-ray fluoroscopy, K-wire drivers, minor procedure operating rooms with field sterility, and hand therapists on site. Hand trauma seen in the emergency department in daytime hours is funneled directly to the wide-awake local anesthesia no tourniquet technique (WALANT) surgery center next door, where there is a plastic surgeon working every day doing minor hand procedures, like carpal tunnel surgery or trauma, from the evening or night before. The hand trauma is inserted into the schedule as it arrives and dealt with expeditiously without going to the main operating room. The patient sees hand therapists before, during, and after the surgery, and then is discharged home right after trauma treatment.

CALGARY

In 1969, Dr Dale Birdsell pioneered wide-awake hand surgery outside of the main operating room in Calgary when he started practice after fellowships at Johns Hopkins and Stanford. The high volume of work and shortage of general anesthesia time in the main operating room pressured the

new approach. This rapidly became the standard of care in Calgary with a very organized trauma management system outside of the main operating room. All hospitals in that city now even have a weekend day shift nurse on duty in minor procedure clinic operating rooms outside the main operating room. The nurse helps the hand surgeon perform hand trauma surgery with field sterility not only on weekends, but also during every week day. Very little of Calgary's minor hand trauma surgery has gone to the main operating room in that city of 1.6 million people for the past 50 years.

Many other hospitals in most Canadian cities have followed a path similar to Calgary and Ottawa. The remainder of this article focuses on Saint John, Winnipeg, and Halifax, which have all developed WALANT hand surgery outside the main operating room at different speeds.

SAINT JOHN

As in the rest of Canada, most of the hand surgery in Saint John is performed by plastic surgeons. McGill-trained Dr Johan Cornelis was the first plastic surgeon in New Brunswick in Saint John in 1968. Like most plastic surgeons, he excised skin cancer in the clinic minor procedure rooms with field sterility outside the main operating room from the beginning. Most North American plastic surgeons have also removed most skin cancers in minor procedure rooms with field sterility, as have the dermatologists, with very acceptable infection rates.[6] The same field sterility principles are applied to laceration repair in emergency departments. The concept of operating outside the main operating room with field sterility has therefore always been very acceptable in Canada.

In 1983, the new Saint John Regional Hospital was built with 2 well-equipped minor procedure rooms in the clinic where field sterility procedures, such as skin cancers, could be easily booked and performed by a plastic surgeon and 1 nurse to assist and circulate as required. Carpal tunnel and trigger finger surgery were still performed in the main operating room at that time, but without sedation. The new hospital was wisely built with more operating theater rooms than was required. As a result, Saint John surgeons had ready access to local anesthesia time in main operating room theaters without anesthesiologists. The surgeons injected the local anesthesia for the hand surgery in the main operating room just as they did for the skin cancers in the clinics. However, tourniquets were used for carpal tunnel surgery until we started using epinephrine in carpal tunnels in the late 1980s.

In the 1990s, Drs Gerry Sparkes, Jim O'Brien, and Don Lalonde moved all of the WALANT trigger finger and carpal tunnel surgery outside the main operating room into the clinic minor procedure rooms, as they were not much different in difficulty or time requirement than skin cancers, especially after eliminating the tourniquet. The hospital would not buy a low-power X-ray fluoroscopy machine to permit moving finger fractures out of the main operating room. Fortunately, Dr Lalonde was able to get the Ladies' Auxiliary Charity organization to buy a fluoroscope for the clinic. That and a battery-operated K-wire driver enabled us to move most of the rest of the minor hand surgery procedures out of the main operating room by 2001. That was also the year that Keith Denkler published his seminal article on lidocaine and epinephrine safety in the finger.[7] Those 2 events saw Saint John start to use lidocaine and epinephrine for most finger and hand operations with field sterility outside of the main operating rooms. Patients now referred to the hand surgery clinic from the emergency department usually undergo any required surgical intervention on Mondays, Tuesdays, Thursdays, and Fridays in daytime hours. This eliminated the previous situation of having to admit patients to hospital beds for main operating room surgery that frequently happened in the evening or night after days of delay.

Saint John went on to publish a multicenter prospective study of more than 1504 patients that proved that field sterility for carpal tunnel surgery is performed with a very low acceptable infection rate of 0.39%.[8] All 6 cases of infection of the study were only superficial and responded to oral or no antibiotics. None of the cases required intravenous antibiotics, incision and drainage, or hospitalization.

The message for surgeons pioneering WALANT trauma in their centers is to get a charitable organization to purchase a K-wire driver and a low-power Fluoroscan X-Ray machine if the hospital will not see the wisdom of doing this. Those are the main 2 things that are required to start WALANT trauma hand surgery outside the main operating room.

The Saint John Regional Hospital had hand therapists in their department in a different area of the hospital from the location of the minor procedure rooms from the beginning in 1983. In the mid-1980s, Dr Gerry Sparkes convinced the hospital administration that we could provide better hand trauma care if we could have 1 hand therapist come to our plastic surgery clinic to see hand trauma with us for 2 hours every Monday morning. This would allow surgeons and therapists to see patients together for better planning and communication. Over the years, this has progressed to the point where we have up to 3 hand therapists up to 4 mornings a week working with the hand surgeons in the hand surgery clinic in 2018. The hand therapists see patients, take over care of minor hand trauma, remove sutures, build splints, and educate patients with hand trauma before, during, and after their surgery in the clinic. In the case of flexor tendon repairs and finger fracture K wiring, hand therapists come into the clinic operating room to see the repairs while the patients actively move their fingers during the surgery. Patients see that therapists are part of the team. Patients see therapists interact with the surgeons. Surgeons, therapists, and patients all discuss postoperative management during the surgery.

The integration of clinic-based hand surgery with hand therapy allows better communication among the surgeon, patient, and therapist to decrease the possibility of postoperative complications. It also decreases the number of required visits for the patient and ensures that therapy is initiated in a timely manner.

WINNIPEG

Clinic-based hand surgery can have a variety of interpretations depending on the degree of adoption within the institution. Winnipeg is a good example of one of the later adopters of the system described for Calgary, Ottawa, and Saint John with more and more procedures moving out of the main operating room and into a clinic-based setting over the past 10 years. As the tertiary referral center for Manitoba (drawing a population of 1.2 million) in a very large geographic region, hand surgery delivery has evolved in Winnipeg.

Ten years ago, elective hand surgery, including carpal tunnel, trigger finger, and some Dupuytren excision, took place under WALANT in minor procedure operating rooms with skin cancer excisions. For hand trauma, patients would have minor procedures, such as extensor tendon repairs or fracture reductions, performed in the emergency department with field sterility. Patients needing K-wire fixation, flexor tendon repair, and more extensive explorations would be held in the emergency department and booked for main operating room full sterility surgery.

A main force for change came from overcrowding of the emergency department. This constraint is not unique to Winnipeg or even Canadian centers. Moving minor hand surgery to clinics solved the problem. In Winnipeg, the overcrowding problem led to the development decanting clinic, where minor procedures are now performed. For the emergency room, it allowed faster patient discharge. For the hand surgery team, it allowed more efficient management of these patients with dedicated nursing staff and supplies. For the patients, it provided a much more pleasant and efficient environment than the main operating room or the emergency department.

In the past 10 years, the capacity of the decanting hand surgery clinic to perform more complex trauma in the clinic has expanded. All manner of traumatic reconstructions are now regularly performed, including K-wire fracture fixation, and flexor tendon and nerve repair. If surgery is delayed, it is usually completed within 1 to 2 days during a booked time in the clinic. Before implementing this care model, some patients would wait 1 to 2 weeks for main operating room time to become available. Offloading most patients with hand trauma from the main operating room not only decreases the costs to the health care system, it also frees main operating room time for more complex cases. Most hand trauma patients in Winnipeg now bypass the emergency room and are triaged directly to the hand surgery clinic. The volume of patients seen averages more than 3000 per year, with roughly one-third of those requiring surgery. After assessment, most patients are provided with definitive treatment the same day.

The Impact of Clinic Wide-Awake Local Anesthesia No Tourniquet Technique on Finances and Quality of Life in Winnipeg

The impact of this transition to clinic-based surgery has been a decrease in surgical wait times, increased surgeon convenience, and significant cost savings for the main operating room and the hospital, as well as the Canadian taxpayers who fund all health care in Canada.

There are several financial and patient care benefits arising from a dedicated hand surgery clinic with procedural capabilities. With costs for main operating room time estimated at $36 to $37 per minute, even simple procedures can incur substantial costs.[9] Costs for clinic-based procedures are usually limited to equipment processing and expendable items, and therefore offer a large cost reduction. In Winnipeg, in the last 6 months before this writing, more than 160 patients requiring flexor tendon repair or K-wire fixation have had their surgeries performed outside of the main operating room in our hand surgery clinic with WALANT. Using a very conservative estimate of 1 hour of main operating room time saved per case, the cost savings are more than $350,000. In practice, these savings are not truly realized in the main operating room budget, as other cases inevitably fill the available operating time. For this reason, requests for clinic funding are best made

to administrators who are responsible for health care funding at a higher level than administrators concerned only about main operating room budgets. We have found both hospital and health region executive officers to be very receptive to funding requests when presented with our cost savings data.

In Winnipeg, patients routinely travel hundreds of miles from rural and northern locations to obtain consultation for hand surgery and traumatic injuries. Offering expedited surgery has significant implications for these patients. Before implementing our hand surgery clinic, patients placed on the main operating room emergency waiting list not only had to fast to get sedation, but they had to either occupy a hospital bed or secure and pay lodging to be available on short notice to get into the main operating room. This had a significant negative financial impact on patients. It reduced their quality of life and their ability to work while awaiting surgery. Also, many of these patients were from vulnerable populations who were unable to get lodging or come back to the hospital. Surgical delays would often lead to missed operating room dates, loss to follow-up, and poor outcomes.

In Winnipeg, as in the rest of Canada, main operating room hand surgery typically occurred after daytime hours and with unpredictable timing. In the summer peak trauma season, backlogs led to elective slate cancellation to facilitate timely completion of emergency cases. Following implementation of our hand surgery clinic, these inconveniences were eliminated. It is now rare for our staff to operate after daytime hours on nonurgent hand surgery cases, as nearly all cases are performed during our scheduled daytime clinic.

Another benefit to our hand surgeons and patients is that there is a decreased need to assess and treat patients in the emergency department after hours. The resources and assistance available in this setting can often be lacking, especially if a procedure is required. Treatment of these patients can instead be diverted to a daytime clinic with appropriate lighting, equipment, and rested personnel to assist with the procedures. With multiple rooms available for patient assessments, high-volume centers, such as Winnipeg, can efficiently manage their trauma consults during daytime hours.

What Does the Clinic-Based Surgery Center in Winnipeg Look Like?

Obstacles to developing a clinic-based hand surgery program include getting the required space and initial investment in equipment. In Winnipeg, a decommissioned patient ward used for follow-up clinics was repurposed into an emergency patient decanting hand surgery clinic with minor procedure rooms. The first iteration of this clinic was implemented with only basic equipment obtained from hospital surplus at no cost (**Fig. 1**). A stretcher, portable light, and hand table (repurposed patient tray) were placed in each of 4 rooms. Portable carts with sutures, local anesthetic, dressing supplies, and basic instruments were also available along with a splinting cart. Although far from fully equipped, this basic setup allowed for a successful proof of concept and further development of the clinic.

Initially, instrument sets matching what was available in the operating room were used. These proved to be expensive and had too many unnecessary instruments for most of our clinic procedures. We subsequently created simple hand instrument trays tailored for this setting that are comprehensive yet minimalistic to reduce costs and allow for greater availability (**Fig. 2**). These sets contain a Freer elevator, Senn retractors, skin hooks, tenotomy and iris scissors, mosquito forceps, toothed Adson forceps, small Adson self-retaining retractor, and cutting and standard needle drivers. Access to an electrocautery unit can be useful, but we have found that for most cases this is not required. All of our cases are performed with epinephrine without the use of tourniquet and we do not consider cautery to be a requirement for clinic-based hand surgery. With

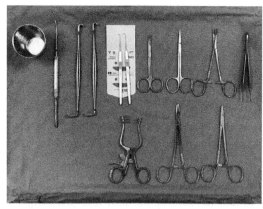

Fig. 2. Hand tray used for most clinic-based hand surgeries in Winnipeg. From top left: Freer elevator, Senn retractors, skin hooks, tenotomy and iris scissors, mosquito forceps, toothed Adson forceps, small Adson self-retaining retractor, and cutting and standard needle driver.

even this limited equipment, most elective and traumatic soft tissue cases can be performed with ease.

To increase our capabilities, we added fracture fixation equipment with a mini low-power X-ray C-arm and K-wire driver. Our current instruments are a Fluoroscan (InSight FD; Hologic, Marlborough, MA) C-arm and battery-powered wire drivers (CD8; Stryker, Kalamazoo, MI). Far more basic equipment setups have been safely used for wire fixation.[10] We also now have computer access to the hospital radiograph system to see images taken in the emergency department.

Recently an operative microscope has been added to our clinic and has been used in nerve repair. Proximal nerve blocks can be helpful in these cases. Alternatively, the proximal nerve stumps of larger lacerated nerves can be visualized and small needles (30 gauge) can infiltrate lidocaine and epinephrine into the epineurium under direct vision. We have found that access to ultrasound equipment has helped regional anesthetic techniques for proximal nerve blocks. These blocks are usually performed at the level of the elbow or proximal forearm using techniques well described in the literature.[11] Our experience is that most learners with basic ultrasound training can quickly become successful with these techniques. Proximal ultrasound-guided nerve blocks also can be helpful in the fixation of multiple metacarpal fractures and in repairing injuries in multiple digits. Epinephrine still needs to be injected with lidocaine in the operative field if hemostasis is important. Proximal nerve blocks create a distal sympathectomy and more bleeding in surgery without a tourniquet.

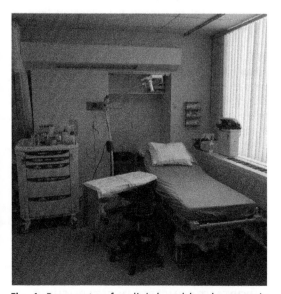

Fig. 1. Room setup for clinic-based hand surgery in Winnipeg. This is a repurposed patient ward room. Basic requirements include adjustable stretcher and hand table, portable light, and equipment cart. The same room can be used for K-wire insertion with fluoroscopy, with the hand table being replaced by a mini C-arm.

The small size of modern fluoroscopic low-power C-arm units makes their use feasible, in even small clinic rooms. Battery-powered K-wire and drill systems eliminate the need for space-occupying power sources and extraneous cables that can impair movement in small rooms and lead to inadvertent contamination of the sterile field. Our clinic procedure rooms are 9 by 12 feet in dimension and provide ample space even with an assistant and nurse. For most cases, including all soft tissue procedures, draping is performed with 4 small green towels. When fluoroscopy is used, a small split sheet is used to allow greater freedom for moving the arm and obtaining the required views. Safe infection rates have been documented with K-wire insertion performed with field sterility.[12] Wide-awake approaches have been shown to be effective and well tolerated for plate-and-screw fixation in the hand.[13,14]

Availability of a space with multiple rooms is one of the most crucial factors in determining overall efficiency in clinic-based hand surgery. With 3 to 4 treatment rooms, multiple patients can be assessed and given local anesthetic in a short time. The surgeon or assistant can inject local anesthesia in one patient and then continue with the next patient assessment or surgery while that local anesthetic and epinephrine take maximal effect. If multiple rooms are not available, patients can be injected with local anesthetic and then moved to the waiting room to free up space.

Transitioning between models of care delivery can be difficult, especially when the funding for the main operating room is managed separately from funding for the clinic. For those working within a block-funding health care model, these savings offer a real benefit to the system and all the stakeholders. For those within a more traditional funding by department model, instituting change may be more difficult. The philosophy behind the Winnipeg clinic development was to keep costs low in the beginning and demonstrate utility. The initial funding for this clinic came from the follow-up clinic budget located in the same hospital unit. This proof of concept was a powerful tool that allowed the hand surgeons to advocate for increased resources from the overall hospital administration. Not only was the clinic well received and subsequently better funded, it was used as a model for other surgical departments looking to offload their consults from the emergency department.

Improved Surgical Education

Limited main operating room access to time places limits on the amount of time that can be allotted to resident education. This also means decreased operating time for residents and limited teaching time during cases to follow rigid main operating room time schedules.

The increased availability and flexibility of time allowed by a clinic-based procedure room has helped to eliminate these problems. Our residents can do more cases at a more relaxed supervised pace without a tourniquet. In Winnipeg, our current setup has the residents running a trauma clinic supervised by a hand surgeon. The residents consent the patient, inject the local anesthesia, and perform the surgery with the assistance of the attending surgeon. With more operating room time available for complex cases and less room turnover time, teaching and resident participation has increased. Feedback from our training program has been very positive from both the residents and attending surgeons.

HALIFAX

Halifax, another regional referral center in Canada, is progressing along the same path to developing a wide-awake hand surgery center, but it is just beginning to move trauma hand surgery out of the main operating room. Currently the hand surgery service has access to 2 days per week for emergency procedures in the main operating room with full sterility, tourniquet surgery, and sedation. However, it is not uncommon for the emergency list to exceed the allocated time. In response, the surgeons have repurposed a previously underutilized minor procedure room for WALANT placement of K-wires, as well as other small hand surgery cases. They have just begun wide-awake flexor tendon repair in that city. A surplus high-power mini C-arm was obtained from the main operating room, and K-wire drivers were made available. The relatively small addition of equipment to the existing minor surgery clinic has dramatically increased the types of hand cases that can be performed outside of the main operating room, at a minimal cost to the system. Although this model does not yet allow for the same efficiency of patient flow as in Winnipeg, Saint John, Calgary, and Ottawa, it helps prove the concept to the administration and provides an inroad to further development.

IMPORTANT CONCEPTS IN ESTABLISHING WIDE-AWAKE LOCAL ANESTHESIA NO TOURNIQUET HAND SURGERY OUTSIDE THE MAIN OPERATING ROOM

- Existing resources such as a clinic, minor procedure room, or unused hospital rooms should provide the starting point for moving cases from the main operating room.

- Required instrumentation can often be obtained from surplus or borrowed equipment from the main operating room.
- The initial goal is to provide a minimally expensive proof of concept to demonstrate to the administration and personnel the benefits of the WALANT care model outside of the main operating room.
- Surgeons should start with simple procedures and progress to more complex cases as their comfort with WALANT increases.
- Demonstrate safe evidence-based field sterility literature to the administration, as well as the safety record of established Canadian WALANT sites.
- Educate administrators about the financial benefits of moving minor hand surgery out of the main operating room.
- Get external funding if necessary to obtain a low-power fluoroscopic radiograph machine and a K-wire driver.
- Educate nurses and administrators about the increased safety of surgery when sedation is eliminated.
- Advocate change on behalf of your patients to increase the convenience and safety of their surgery while reducing their costs and the unnecessary garbage production detrimental to our environment.

With this care model becoming the standard of care in multiple centers across Canada, the argument for its value is becoming less and less difficult.

REFERENCES

1. Nodwell T, Lalonde DH. How long does it take phentolamine to reverse adrenaline-induced vasoconstriction in the finger and hand? A prospective randomized blinded study: the Dalhousie project experimental phase. Can J Plast Surg 2003;11: 187–90.
2. Lalonde D, Bell M, Benoit P, et al. A multicenter prospective study of 3,110 consecutive cases of elective epinephrine use in the fingers and hand: the Dalhousie Project clinical phase. J Hand Surg Am 2005;30:1061–7.
3. Chowdhry S, Seidenstricker L, Cooney DS, et al. Do not use epinephrine in digital blocks: myth or truth? Part II. A retrospective review of 1111 cases. Plast Reconstr Surg 2010;126:2031–4.
4. Fitzcharles-Bowe C, Denkler K, Lalonde D. Finger injection with high-dose (1:1,000) epinephrine: Does it cause finger necrosis and should it be treated? Hand (N Y) 2007;2:5–11.
5. Thomson CJ, Lalonde DH, Denkler KA, et al. A critical look at the evidence for and against elective epinephrine use in the finger. Plast Reconstr Surg 2007;119:260–6.
6. Alam M, Ibrahim O, Nodzenski M, et al. Adverse events associated with mohs micrographic surgery: multicenter prospective cohort study of 20,821 cases at 23 centers. JAMA Dermatol 2013;149: 1378–85.
7. Denkler K. A comprehensive review of epinephrine in the finger: to do or not to do. Plast Reconstr Surg 2001;08:114–24.
8. Leblanc MR, Lalonde DH, Thoma A, et al. Is main operating room sterility really necessary in carpal tunnel surgery? A multicenter prospective study of minor procedure room field sterility surgery. Hand (N Y) 2011;6:60–3.
9. Childers CP, Maggard-Gibbons M. Understanding costs of care in the operating room. JAMA Surg 2018;153:e176233.
10. Bell M. Emergency finger fractures–an easy fix. Can J Plast Surg 2007;15:179.
11. Milligan R, Houmes S, Goldberg LC, et al. Ultrasound-guided forearm nerve blocks in managing hand and finger injuries. Intern Emerg Med 2017; 12:381–5.
12. Starker I, Eaton RG. Kirschner wire placement in the emergency room. Is there a risk? J Hand Surg Br 1995;20:535–8.
13. Gong KT, Xing SG. How to establish and standardize wide-awake hand surgery: experience from China. J Hand Surg Eur Vol 2017;42:868–70.
14. Xing SG, Tang JB. Surgical treatment, hardware removal, and the wide-awake approach for metacarpal fractures. Clin Plast Surg 2014;41:463–80.

Impact of Wide-Awake Local Anesthesia No Tourniquet on Departmental Settings, Cost, Patient and Surgeon Satisfaction, and Beyond

Jin Bo Tang, MD[a],*, Shu Guo Xing, MD[a],
Egemen Ayhan, MD[b], Sebastian Hediger, MD[c],
Simon Huang, FRCSEd (Plast)[d]

KEYWORDS

- Local anesthesia • No tourniquet • Hand surgery • Efficiency • Departmental settings
- Medical cost • Quality of life • Hand surgery training

KEY POINTS

- The impact of wide-awake hand surgery without tourniquet has started to reveal itself, which includes more efficient departmental settings and savings patients' medical cost, and efficiency of fellowship training and practice of junior hand surgeons.
- The medical cost of the commonly performed procedures is decreased remarkably with WALANT. The cost of a carpal tunnel release with WALANT is only one-third that with brachial plexus block in China.
- Efficiency of fellowship training and practice of junior surgeons are benefited from this approach in 2 units in Turkey and Switzerland, with remarkable savings in medical cost in those patients in Switzerland.
- Overall, this approach improves the surgeons' and patients' quality of life. The improved efficiency lessens the rate of performing surgery in the late afternoon or in the night.

The impact of wide-awake hand surgery without tourniquet has started to reveal itself. Because of differences in cultural background, training systems, health care (insurance) systems and disease distribution, the impact of this new technique is different in each country. We understand that presentation of the wide varieties of changes with this technique in all or many countries worldwide is challenging. In this article, the authors summarize the impact of this new technique in 3 countries in 3 geographic regions on departmental settings, medical cost, patient and surgeon satisfaction, as well as hand surgery training. The 3 countries are China, Turkey, and Switzerland, located in

[a] Department of Hand Surgery, Affiliated Hospital of Nantong University, 20 West Temple Road, Nantong 226001, Jiangsu, China; [b] Hand Surgery, Orthopaedics and Traumatology, University of Health Sciences, Diskapi Yildirim Beyazit Training and Research Hospital, Altındag, Ankara 06110, Turkey; [c] Department of Hand Surgery, Bülach Hospital, Rodenbergstrasse 4, Diessenhofen 8253, Switzerland; [d] Chirurgie Lindenpark, Surgical Day Case Center, Lindenstrasse 23, Kloten 8302, Switzerland
* Corresponding author.
E-mail address: jinbotang@yahoo.com

Hand Clin 35 (2019) 29–34
https://doi.org/10.1016/j.hcl.2018.08.012
0749-0712/19/© 2018 Elsevier Inc. All rights reserved.

East Asia, West Asia bordering Europe, and in the middle continental Europe, respectively.

IMPACT ON DEPARTMENTAL SETTINGS AND PATIENTS' MEDICAL COST IN NANTONG, CHINA

Departmental Settings and Efficiency of Patient Care

In Nantong, China, all levels of hand surgeons in the department of the Nantong University hospital have a great enthusiasm for this technique. The department chairperson has been making the required changes in the organization to adopt tourniquet-free surgery to increase the efficiency and comfort of patient care. A wide-awake hand surgical operating room was built within the hand surgery department outside of the main operating room in the hospital for this new hand surgery approach. As a result of such a change, the wide-awake surgical theater now handles approximately 1 of 6 of the operative cases of the department. This facility accommodated 722 patients in the past year. This accounts for 60% of the all patients operated with the wide-awake method in this department, with the other 40% of wide-awake local anesthesia no tourniquet (WALANT) operations happening in the main operating rooms (**Table 1**). This has efficiently off-loaded the pressure on the 4 main operating rooms that have served the department for nearly 2 decades.

The lack of anesthesiologist requirement and locating the new wide-awake operating room close to the doctors' offices, have resulted in a huge saving in doctors' and patients' time. The surgery can be scheduled whenever the room is free. Patients can be operated the same day they are seen in clinic and the day they decide to have surgery. For doctors, no booking or waiting time is necessary, which is a great preoperative time saver. Establishment of this surgical theater almost completely abolishes the need to perform the surgery in the late afternoon or even in evening in the major operating theater. This improves the surgeons' and patients' quality of life. The surgeons in the team feel their life has been changed for the better. The detail of location of this facility in the department was described in a previous review.[1] The benefits of such a facility are continuing to reveal themselves. The transformation has been remarkable.

Patients' Medical Cost

An audit in April of 2018, on patients who had carpal tunnel release procedures (n = 52) under local anesthesia and those who had same surgery under brachial plexus anesthesia (n = 16) indicates that the total medical cost (including surgical cost, anesthesia, material cost, and so on) of a carpal tunnel release under local anesthesia is only one-third of that under brachial plexus block. The cost for local anesthesia was an average of RMB 114 Yuan for a patient as compared with an average of RMB 2429 Yuan for having a brachial plexus block. It is worth mentioning that patients who get a brachial plexus block in our hospitals traditionally do not get sedation as they do in the West, so that cost is not even in there. The surgical theater's occupying time of a wide-awake carpal tunnel release is two-thirds of that under brachial plexus block. This means a considerable cost-saving for the patient and health care insurance for the country as well as an improvement of efficiency by using one-third less time in the operating room.

Surgeons' Time-Saving

The surgeon's time consumed for each patient is difficult to quantify. The great simplicity of scheduling cases is a great surgeon time saver. Minimal turnover time in the operating room is also a major time saver. Immediate allocation of the patients for

Table 1
Distribution of hand surgery procedures in the wide-awake operating theater and 4 hand surgery main operating rooms in Nantong University, Jiangsu, China

Facilities	Wide-Awake Only Theater	Main Hand Surgery Operating Room
Number of rooms	1	4
Case numbers (yearly)	700–900	3000–3500 (total)
WALANT	All	15%–20% of the cases
Anesthesiologist	Not available	Always available
Nurses in room	One nurse always available	Nurse team always available
Locations	Within department	Adjacent to department, side by side
Distance (doctors' offices)	<5–20 m	From 20–80 m

surgery in an operative facility that only requires decisions and directions from the surgeons is a huge saving of administrative time. The surgeons' willingness to adopt this technique is perhaps mostly because this approach saves so much surgeon time.

The experience of hand surgeons in Tianjin Hospital of China echo the findings in Nantong.[2] In that hospital, a total of 7673 patients were operated with this approach. Besides savings in medical cost, minimal turnover in emergency hand trauma cases and convenience and efficiency of the doctors are the major reasons of their adoption of this method. All their department members like this new approach.[2] Similar to the findings of recent reports,[3,4] the medical cost was remarkably decreased and no increase in infection rate was found. In other hospitals in China, surgeries on flexor and extensor tendons and facture fixation previously done under brachial plexus anesthesia[5,6] are increasingly performed under this new approach. The surgeons in Nantong are moving toward performing flap transfers in the hand using this approach.[7] Although they did not use it in digital replantation, as some other surgeons do,[8] they consider flap harvest generally safe with this approach.

IMPACT ON PRACTICE OF JUNIOR HAND SURGEONS IN ANKARA, TURKEY

When Egemen Ayhan was a fellowship trainee in a busy tertiary referral hospital in Hand Surgery Division, Orthopedics and Traumatology, Mersin University Faculty of Medicine, Mersin, Turkey, Bier block (intravenous regional anesthesia) was a common way of anesthesia for surgeries for hand trauma in the main operating room. At the end of his fellowship before June 2016, he started to perform the WALANT approach and was impressed by its efficiency in several trauma cases.

After his fellowship training, he moved to a hospital in Ankara in June 2016 for hand surgery compulsory health service, which is required in his country before starting to work as a hand surgery specialist. It was difficult for Dr Ayhan to get main operating room time. However, he was offered an everyday-ready minor procedure room outside of the main operating room without anesthesiologist availability. That was the tipping point for him to use the WALANT approach in hand surgery procedures. He clearly benefited from this approach because he performed 502 WALANT procedures with this approach during his first 20-month work as a junior hand surgeon from June 2016 to March 2018 (**Table 2**). Similarly, one of

his colleagues performed more than 150 procedures with this approach during his 1-year fellowship. They both feel that WALANT provides a great opportunity for trainees to perform more cases in a much simpler surgical setting.

Later in the period of his compulsory health service, his hospital offered Egemen Ayhan 2 days a week in the main operating room with general anesthesia availability. He chose to continue to perform some of the procedures with WALANT in the main operating room. His experience in compulsory health service as a junior hand surgeon indicates that WALANT is a very practical and time-saving approach for an intensive workload.

An even more important reason to use WALANT was to have the opportunity to evaluate intraoperative active movement of the hand.[9–14] In his trauma cases (tendon-related procedures, phalangeal and metacarpal fractures), he enjoyed observing the active movement together with the patients. After tendon repairs, he could evaluate the gliding of tendons, the tension of the repair, and any gap formation. Similarly, after surgical fixation of phalangeal and metacarpal fractures, he

Table 2 The procedures performed with WALANT approach in Diskapi Yildirim Beyazit Training and Research Hospital in Ankara, Turkey, in 2016	
Surgical Procedures	**Patients (n = 502)**
Removal of soft tissue tumors (dorsal wrist ganglions, flexor sheath ganglions, giant cell tendon sheath tumors, lipomas, neuromas)	124
Trigger finger release	117
Tendon surgery (repairs, transfers, or tenolysis)	72
Carpal tunnel release	70
Foreign body and implant extraction	41
Local finger flaps and finger or ray amputations	20
Phalangeal fracture fixation and ligament repair	19
Metacarpal fracture fixation	13
Nerve repairs	12
De Quervain release or lateral epicondylitis release	8
Cubital tunnel release or Guyon canal release	4
Dupuytren contracture	2

could check the rotation of the digits and stability of the fixation by active movement of the digits and the hand. He could make intraoperative adjustments that he and the patients could see would improve the final results.

IMPACT ON TREATMENT IN EMERGENCY SETTINGS, TACKLING RESTRICTIONS IN TRAINING AND MEDICAL COST IN BÜLACH ZH, SWITZERLAND
The Use in Emergency Settings and by Trainees

Between April 2016 and April 2017, Sebastian Hediger was a trainee in the role of performing surgeon. He and his surgical supervisor/mentor, who acted as his surgical assistant, performed surgery using WALANT on 29 consecutive trauma and 24 elective surgery patients at a regional hospital in Bülach ZH, Switzerland. Thirteen patients had foreign body removal. There were 11 tendon repairs, 10 carpal tunnel releases, 7 excisional biopsies of benign tumors, 5 nerve repairs, 4 trigger finger releases, 2 ligament repairs, and 1 repair of a "spaghetti wrist." Although the elective WALANT cases took place in the main operating room, the focus of the following paragraphs is on the trauma patients (n = 29) treated in the emergency department.

All injuries in the 29 patients were treated without delay within 2 hours after trauma. In a survey by Businger and colleagues,[15] 63% of Swiss surgical residents and 77% of consultants reported a negative effect on surgical training mainly due to reduced operating room time as a consequence of the 50-hour work time restriction in Switzerland as implemented in 2005. WALANT has a benefit that helps to successfully tackle these restrictions. This method can be implemented as a perfectly suitable teaching tool for junior hand surgeons, which generates and teaches a degree of autonomy to the trainee.

The need for an anesthesiologist, additional staff, and the extensive infrastructure of an operating room is eliminated. They scheduled these cases mostly in-between regular consultation hours, sometimes during the lunch hour, or just after the daily schedule. In most cases, this led to a perfect integration of these operations into the working day and provided ample additional training time. The 50-hour working week limit was not breached. WALANT created much needed additional educational or instructional operating time.

They injected a 50:50 mixture of ropivacaine 1% and lidocaine 1% with epinephrine for all cases. This ensured a rapid onset and a prolonged anesthetic effect. Sufficient postoperative analgesia was thereby achieved, yet optimal conditions for operations beyond 5 hours if required.

WALANT greatly reduces time pressure for the trainee hand surgeon. A stress-free, tourniquet-free learning environment is created in which time-consuming instructional advice can take place in a relaxed atmosphere. This in itself improves the quality of training because the trainee's and trainer's surgical performance is improved by limiting the stressor of time pressure.[16,17] This is even more evident when the procedures are performed outside of the main operating room environment.

In the main operating room, additional time pressures regularly occur by newly booked urgent cases. WALANT bypasses this and many other resource constraints and allows the trainee hand surgeon to create his or her own timetable. The trainee hand surgeon and his or her trainer do not need to wait for a free operating slot. By bypassing such resource constraints, it can be clearly seen that educational operating time for the trainee schedule can be created with a multi-advantageous ease when using a WALANT approach.

Their experience showed that professional and transparent communication about the educational setup of the operation was never encountered with mistrust by the patient with regard to being treated by a trainee. The patients gained the impression that the wide-awake setting helped create a safe, positive, satisfactory learning environment for all involved. The transparent communication enhanced the patients' understanding of the procedure and the possible difficult phases, thus increasing the awareness of the degree of injury and the later required rehabilitation.

It is worth mentioning that some patients, such as those with high anxiety or young age, might not tolerate the transparent surgical setting and the wide-awake approach.

Cost Savings

The 29 patients in Bülach ZH treated by 2 authors (SHediger and SHuang) demonstrates a reduction in overall treatment cost by 49%. The non-WALANT traditional approach usually involves more costly intravenous regional anesthesia or plexus anesthesia in the operating room. A recent publication by Rhee and colleagues[3] showed even more extensive cost savings for the US Military Health Care System for comparable hand surgery procedures ranging from 70% to 85%. Leblanc and colleagues[18] concluded in their detailed cost analysis for carpal tunnel surgery that using the main operating room is almost 4 times more expensive than an ambulatory setting. The Swiss calculations are based on TARMED, the standard Swiss tariff for outpatient services. They considered mean values of their patient group and included anesthesia, surgery, and material costs, as well as use of the operating room and nonphysician care. In the 29 patients, a total of nearly 35,000 Swiss francs (roughly $36,000 US) were saved.

Many things make the use of WALANT highly cost-effective. These points are specific for the Swiss health care system, but at least some of these should be applicable internationally:

- The Swiss health care system financially compensates a day-case surgical procedure with a defined fixed tariff (based on the "TARMED" system). In addition, there can be an anesthesiologist's fee, which is left out when a WALANT approach is applied. Thus, almost 50% of the total costs can be saved in small to medium-priced cases.
- The health care provider can significantly reduce costs within the "TARMED" system, as WALANT allows delivery of a surgical procedure with fewer staff and cost-effective resources/infrastructure.
- With the WALANT method, the administration of local anesthesia is charged by the surgeon. Accordingly, the surgeon's remuneration is usually at a lower level than that of an anesthesiologist.
- An injured patient will receive operative treatment within the budgetary unit of the emergency department, and therefore the cost for the wide-awake approach is at least in part absorbed by the expenditure already generated by the emergency department.

SOME ISSUES IN FURTHER PROMOTING WIDE-AWAKE SURGICAL TECHNIQUES WHERE IT IS NOT YET AVAILABLE
"Epinephrine Fear" Still Exists for Surgeons Who Have Not Kept up with the Literature

Although most surgeons in most countries now accept a minimal risk in using epinephrine in fingers and hand, there endures a hesitation against WALANT in some doctors in some countries. Breaking the epinephrine and digital necrosis myth is still hard work. Almost all older surgeons have learned during medical school education that epinephrine should not be injected into fingers, nose, penis, and toes.[19] This expression reminds us of Albert Einstein's quote: *"It is harder to crack prejudice than an atom."* Acceptance of epinephrine and lidocaine for local anesthesia continues to progress, particularly since the

publication of the multicenter prospective study of 3110 consecutive cases of elective epinephrine use in the fingers and hand with no finger loss and no requirement for phentolamine rescue.[20] The supply of phentolamine (Regitin), which is the rescue agent of epinephrine vasoconstriction is problematic in some countries. It is rarely required with surgical doses of 1:100,000 epinephrine, but should be available for accidental finger injection of 1:1000 epinephrine to prevent ischemic reperfusion pain and neuropraxia. Phentolamine is also available to dentists in Europe and North America as Oraverse.

However, surgeons are changing. WALANT is now discussed at most the hand surgery meetings of most countries of the world today. The scope of application is expanding to almost all hand surgical procedures, including microsurgical procedures and emergency operations.[7,8,21,22] The injection of anesthesia becomes almost pain-free.[23,24]

Premixed Anesthetics Are Not Available in Many Countries

The premixed 1:100,000 or 1:200,000 epinephrine with lidocaine is not commercially available in many countries, including China and Turkey. Surgeons there have to prepare a solution using either 1 mg/1 mL or 0.5 mg/mL epinephrine, and dilute it with lidocaine to obtain 1:100,000 epinephrine. To make 1:100,000 epinephrine in 1% lidocaine, mix 0.1 mL of 1/1000 epinephrine from a 1.0-mL syringe into 10 mL of 1% lidocaine. Mixing epinephrine with lidocaine is a simple process.

Anesthesiologists Battle for Keeping Their Patients

Performing many hand surgery procedures without participation of anesthesiologists is very acceptable in many countries where the patients are many and the anesthesiologists are overburdened. However, in some countries, local anesthesia by the surgeons reduces work desired by anesthesiologists. However, good medicine is about what is best for patients, not best for doctors. This topic is often not discussed, but it is partially responsible for slowing the widespread use of WALANT in some countries.

Lack of Powerful Ways to Spread the Word to Surgeons Who Have Not Heard of This Method

Education is necessary for teaching those surgeons in different countries. It is unfortunate that this technique is the least disseminated to those surgeons who may need it most. Surgeons in developing countries have the least access to education. Their patients are those who can least afford unnecessary general anesthesia and sedation in the main operating room. Extending the education through courses, books, lectures, and personal communication to those surgeons in the countries in which not many surgeons are able to regularly attend international hand conferences is an urgent need. It is our goal to help the world reach them through all possible means of education. A book about WALANT with more than 150 videos is available from Thieme. There is a free education website for hand surgeons and therapists (https://walant.surgery).

REFERENCES

1. Tang JB, Gong KT, Zhu L, et al. Performing hand surgery under local anesthesia without a tourniquet in China. Hand Clin 2017;33:415–24.
2. Gong KT, Xing SG. How to establish and standardize wide-awake hand surgery: experience from China. J Hand Surg Eur Vol 2017;42:868–70.
3. Rhee PC, Fischer MM, Rhee LS, et al. Cost savings and patient experiences of a clinic-based, wide-awake hand surgery program at a military medical center: a critical analysis of the first 100 procedures. J Hand Surg Am 2017;42:e139–47.
4. Jagodzinski NA, Ibish S, Furniss D. Surgical site infection after hand surgery outside the operating theatre: a systematic review. J Hand Surg Eur Vol 2017;42:289–94.
5. Zhou X, Li XR, Qing J, et al. Outcomes of the six-strand M-Tang repair for zone 2 primary flexor tendon repair in 54 fingers. J Hand Surg Eur Vol 2017;42:462–8.
6. Pan ZJ, Qin J, Zhou X, et al. Robust thumb flexor tendon repairs with a six-strand M-Tang method, pulley venting, and early active motion. J Hand Surg Eur Vol 2017;42:909–14.
7. Xing SG, Mao T. The use of local anaesthesia with epinephrine in the harvest and transfer of an extended Segmuller flap in the fingers. J Hand Surg Eur Vol 2018;43:783–4.
8. Wong J, Lin CH, Chang NJ, et al. Digital revascularization and replantation using the wide-awake hand surgery technique. J Hand Surg Eur Vol 2017;42:621–5.
9. Lalonde DH, Martin AL. Wide-awake flexor tendon repair and early tendon mobilization in zones 1 and 2. Hand Clin 2013;29:207–13.
10. Higgins A, Lalonde DH, Bell M, et al. Avoiding flexor tendon repair rupture with intraoperative total active movement examination. Plast Reconstr Surg 2010; 126:941–5.
11. Tang JB. Recent evolutions in flexor tendon repairs and rehabilitation. J Hand Surg Eur Vol 2018;43: 469–73.
12. Tang JB. New developments are improving flexor tendon repair. Plast Reconstr Surg 2018;141: 1427–37.
13. Giesen T, Reissner L, Besmens I, et al. Flexor tendon repair in the hand with the M-Tang technique (without peripheral sutures), pulley division, and early active motion. J Hand Surg Eur Vol 2018;43: 474–9.
14. Gregory S, Lalonde DH, Fung Leung LT. Minimally invasive finger fracture management: wide-awake closed reduction, K-wire fixation, and early protected movement. Hand Clin 2014;30:7–15.
15. Businger A, Guller U, Oertli D. Effect of the 50-hour work week limitation on training of surgical residents in Switzerland. Arch Surg 2010;145:558–63.
16. Arora S, Sevdalis N, Nestel D, et al. The impact of stress on surgical performance: a systematic review of the literature. Surgery 2010;147:318–30, 330.e1–6.
17. Wetzel CM, Kneebone RL, Woloshynowych M, et al. The effects of stress on surgical performance. Am J Surg 2006;191:5–10.
18. Leblanc MR, Lalonde J, Lalonde DH. A detailed cost and efficiency analysis of performing carpal tunnel surgery in the main operating room versus the ambulatory setting in Canada. Hand (N Y) 2007;2: 173–8.
19. Bruce AM, Spencer JM. Surgical myths in dermatology. Dermatol Surg 2010;36:512–7.
20. Lalonde D, Bell M, Benoit P, et al. A multicenter prospective study of 3,110 consecutive cases of elective epinephrine use in the fingers and hand: the Dalhousie Project clinical phase. J Hand Surg Am 2005;30:1061–7.
21. Iqbal HJ, Doorgakant A, Rehmatullah NNT, et al. Pain and outcomes of carpal tunnel release under local anaesthetic with or without a tourniquet: a randomized controlled trial. J Hand Surg Eur Vol 2018; 43:808–12.
22. Xing SG, Mao T. Temporary tourniquet use after epinephrine injection to expedite wide awake emergency hand surgeries. J Hand Surg Eur Vol 2018;43: 888–9.
23. Lalonde DH. Conceptual origins, current practice, and views of wide awake hand surgery. J Hand Surg Eur Vol 2017;42:886–95.
24. Lalonde D. Minimally invasive anesthesia in wide awake hand surgery. Hand Clin 2014;30:1–6.

Wide Awake Secondary Tendon Reconstruction

Lin Lin Gao, MD[a],*, James Chang, MD[b]

KEYWORDS

- Two-stage tendon reconstruction • Wide awake • Tenolysis • Local anesthesia • Tendon transfer

KEY POINTS

- The wide awake technique is safe and effective for tenolysis, 2-stage tendon reconstruction, and tendon transfers.
- Modifications to the technique include the use of a short-acting sedative and limited tourniquet time during the initial dissection.
- Using the wide awake technique during tenolysis allows intraoperative identification of adhesions, triggering points, and poor active range of motion, which can be fully addressed during surgery.
- Active flexion and extension are possible under the wide awake technique during the second stage of 2-stage flexor tendon reconstruction. This allows setting appropriate tension, reducing gapping, and preventing tendon imbalances, such as quadriga and the lumbrical-plus deformity.
- The wide awake technique can be used for tendon transfers with better control of clinical outcomes.

 Video content accompanies this article at http://www.hand.theclinics.com/.

INTRODUCTION

Flexor tendon injuries are among the most challenging to manage in hand surgery. Despite improvements in surgical techniques and rehabilitation protocols, restoring full range of motion after tendon injury, especially zone 2 injuries, remains difficult.[1] Flexor tendons and their overlying pulleys are complex structures; both tendon continuity and the ability to glide through the pulley system must be restored. After tendon repair, there are competing demands from immobilization required for optimal tendon healing and the need for early motion to avoid adhesions and stiffness.[1]

Consequently, flexor tendon repair is fraught with complications, including tendon rupture, adhesion formation, joint contracture, triggering, bowstringing, and inaccurate tensioning leading to tendon imbalances.[2] Tendon rupture rates have been reported to be as high as 30%.[3] Stiffness is the most common complication and may be from adhesion formation surrounding the tendon or from joint contracture, which has a reported prevalence of 17%.[4]

Despite optimal surgical technique, some of these complications may be unavoidable, and secondary tendon reconstruction would then be required. Tenolysis may be performed for the stiff digit. Two-stage tendon reconstruction is indicated when flexor tendons and/or the pulley system have been disrupted. Last, if the tendons and muscles are damaged beyond salvage, healthy tendons may be rerouted from the uninjured side for tendon transfers to restore motion.

The recent development of wide awake local anesthesia no tourniquet (WALANT) technique as described by Lalonde has gained increasing

Disclosure Statement: No disclosures.
a Chase Hand and Upper Limb Center, Division of Plastic and Reconstructive Surgery, Stanford University Medical Center, 770 Welch Road, Suite 400, Palo Alto, CA 94304, USA; b Division of Plastic and Reconstructive Surgery, Stanford University Medical Center, 770 Welch Road, Suite 400, Palo Alto, CA 94304, USA
* Corresponding author.
E-mail addresses: llgao@stanford.edu; linlin314@gmail.com

popularity. The WALANT technique has been shown to be a safe, effective, and cost-efficient method that can be applied for many types of hand procedures.[5] In particular, the WALANT technique offers distinct advantages when it is applied to tendon reconstruction.[6] It has become routine for primary flexor tendon repair.[7] Increasingly, it has also been applied with favorable clinical outcomes in secondary tendon reconstruction and tendon transfers.[8]

In this article, the techniques of using wide awake anesthesia as it is applied for tenolysis, 2-stage tendon reconstruction, and tendon transfers are discussed.

INDICATIONS/CONTRAINDICATIONS

Any patient who meets surgical criteria for tenolysis or secondary tendon repair may be a candidate for wide awake anesthesia, with a few exceptions. Children and patients who cannot follow commands are not ideal candidates for wide awake surgery. In addition, those patients with high anxiety who cannot tolerate being awake during surgery are also not appropriate candidates. High vasovagal tone with propensity for loss of consciousness is a relative contraindication. There are described maneuvers that increase cerebral blood flow to minimize loss of consciousness.[9] In extremely rare cases, an allergy to local anesthetics is a contraindication. Allergy to local anesthetics may be due to 2 distinct types: contact dermatitis or swelling from delayed type hypersensitivity (type IV) or anaphylaxis (type I).[10] The incidence of type IV hypersensitivity is reported between 0.7% and 2.4%.[11] The incidence of anaphylaxis in response to amide local anesthetic is extremely rare, and the data are limited to case reports.[12]

During the preoperative clinic visit, the risks and benefits of wide awake tendon repair are discussed with the patient. Appropriate patient selection is essential because some patients may not tolerate being awake in a surgical setting. Because intensive hand therapy is required postoperatively, it is imperative that patients are motivated and understand the rehabilitation process. Noncompliant patients are inappropriate surgical candidates.

SURGICAL TECHNIQUE
General Approach

For many of the secondary tendon reconstruction cases, the standard mixture of 1% lidocaine and 1:100,000 epinephrine as described by Lalonde is preferred with a conservative upper limit of 7 mg/kg.[13] If larger volumes are needed, for example, in the setting of multiple tendon transfers, the standard mixture may be diluted even further into a tumescent solution. There is evidence for lidocaine and epinephrine effectiveness in concentrations as low as 0.2% and 1:1,000,000, respectively.[14] If the procedure length exceeds 2.5 hours, 0.5% bupivacaine with 1:200,000 epinephrine, up to 20 mL, is added.[15]

In the authors' practice at Stanford, several modifications have been made to the classic WALANT technique. All patients are offered monitored anesthesia often in the form of short-acting propofol. The injection is performed under sedation, which delivers a completely pain-free patient experience. During the initial 20 to 30 minutes of dissection, while under sedation, a tourniquet is used to allow for a bloodless field. The tourniquet is released after 20 minutes, at which point the epinephrine has taken full effect. The maximal effect of epinephrine has been shown to occur at 26 minutes and remains effective for 3 to 4 hours.[16] The use of epinephrine cuts down on the inevitable amount of bleeding from the standard WALANT technique. The 20 minutes of tourniquet use do not affect the contractile force of the muscles needed to test active motion later in the operation.

Multiple studies have confirmed the safety of epinephrine use in the digits.[17] However, when performing digital block, it is important to inject only into the subcutaneous tissue and avoid injecting into the sheath. Reports of fingertip necrosis requiring amputation have been described with lidocaine and epinephrine injection into the flexor tendon sheath.[18] In addition, it is essential to ensure the return of blood flow to the digits before patient discharge.[19] If persistent ischemia occurs, reversal with phentolamine is recommended.[18]

Tenolysis

Finger motion is essential for hand function and may be lost most often from traumatic causes.[20] The scar tissue that forms after tendon injury or repair may surround the tendon-pulley interface and may also extend into the joint capsule.[21] Flexor tenolysis is a well-established method to restore motion for stiffness resulting from tendon adhesions, provided that the passive range of motion is greater than the active range of motion.[21] Multiple studies have demonstrated statistically significant improvement in both total passive motion and total active motion after tenolysis.[22] In addition, full release may involve not only releasing the extensor and flexor tendons but also, in the case of limited passive motion, addressing the joint with capsular release, collateral ligament excision, and volar plate release.[23]

It is ideal to wait for a period of 3 to 6 months after tendon repair or grafting to allow soft tissue equilibrium to occur and to ensure maximal range of motion has plateaued with hand therapy.[2] The initial portion of the surgery is performed under tourniquet and sedation. The tendons are exposed and dissected free from any scar and surrounding tissue. Any visible areas of scarring are released. Passive movement of the finger is performed after tenolysis to ensure the joint is mobile. If a joint is involved, capsulotomy is then performed. The excursion is tested by twisting an Allis clamp to avoid any undue tension on the pulleys (Video 1). The sedative is then turned off; the patient awakes, and the tourniquet is deflated. The patient then dynamically ranges his or her fingers and makes a composite fist (Video 2). Any additional tethering points are identified and released, which ensures intraoperatively that the patient has regained full range of motion. The approach to wide awake tenolysis is summarized in Video 3.

Postoperatively, the patient starts early active motion to preserve the range of motion gained during tenolysis. With postoperative swelling and edema that inevitably develop, the range of motion achieved during time of surgery is initially lost, but if the patient is compliant with therapy, it will be regained. Having the patient witness the full range of motion they were able to achieve while in the operating room is a powerful motivator during the ensuing months of hand therapy.

The classic WALANT technique offers several advantages. First, eliminating the tourniquet and its related complications, such as friction burns, ischemia, and pressure-induced muscle damage or neurapraxias, is a clear advantage.[24] The modification of limiting tourniquet time to less than 20 minutes has been shown to be well tolerated.[25] Second, after tenolysis, active patient-initiated motion allows determination of points of additional scarring, which are identified and released. Before, the adequacy of tenolysis could only be determined from passive traction. Third, the strength of the tendon is tested during active movement.[26] Scarred tendon may become frayed, attenuated, and weakened, leading to potential tendon rupture. Poor tendon quality can be identified intraoperatively with active motion, which allows repair or reinforcement with tendon graft, preventing potential tendon rupture.[26] Last, active motion tests the integrity and accommodation of the pulleys. If important pulleys are ruptured during active pull-through, reconstruction or repair is needed. In addition, because the pulley-tendon interface is a common point of adhesion, active motions allow intraoperative balancing with the need to release or vent the pulleys, preventing bowstringing.

Two-Stage Tendon Transfer

Primary flexor tendon repair is not possible in the setting of a highly scarred tissue bed and when the pulley system is damaged. According to the Boyes classification system, primary tendon reconstruction will have suboptimal outcomes when attempted in grade 2 or above[27] (Table 1). Two-stage tendon reconstruction, where a pulley system using silicone rod is created during the first stage, followed by tendon grafting, has been an accepted method of restoring finger flexion.[28]

The indication for 2-stage flexor tendon reconstruction is any severe injury to flexor tendon with loss of the sheath integrity.[29] Joint release and soft tissue coverage may be attempted during the first stage along with creation of the flexor sheath with the silicone rod. Patient selection is critical for successful outcome because the ideal patient is motivated and accepts the long time commitment and extensive hand therapy that are required postoperatively. At the preoperative visit, the importance of rehabilitation and the possibility of less than perfect result are discussed with the patient. Also, the alternatives of accepting the lack of active flexion, tenodesis, and/or joint fusion should be discussed with the patient.

During the first stage, when a silicone rod is placed to re-create the pulley system, a key principle is to perform all the steps such that the second stage involves only passing the tendon graft through the newly reconstructed pulley.[30] This first surgery is usually performed under anesthesia because tensioning is not necessary during this stage (Fig. 1).

The tendon sheath is exposed through a standard Bruner incision. The distal flexor tendon remnants are preserved after flexor digitorum superficialis (FDS) / flexor digitorum profundus (FDP) resection. The silicone rod is sized to approximate the width of the FDP; it is better to select larger rather than smaller size to allow smooth passage of the new tendon graft. The silicone rod is passed beneath the pulley and is sutured distally and left unattached proximally in the wrist/distal forearm. If there are concerns about the integrity of the distal attachment, the rod may be secured via suture button. If the joints are stiff, capsulotomies are performed. If pulley reconstruction is needed, the remnants of the FDS/FDP may used. A2 and A4 pulleys are the most important pulleys to reconstruct to prevent subsequent bowstringing.[31]

Only when the affected fingers have supple joints and achieved soft tissue equilibrium is the second stage of tendon reconstruction appropriate. A minimum of 3 months is needed before the second stage. During this time period, the patient works with therapy to maintain passive full

Table 1
Boyes classification system

Grade 1	Good; supple skin and joints
Grade 2	Scar; heavy scarring of soft tissue
Grade 3	Joint; scarring involves the joint
Grade 4	Artery or nerve; injury involving one or both of neuromuscular bundles
Grade 5	Combination of the above; often severe injury

Data from Boyes JH, Stark HH. Flexor-tendon grafts in the fingers and thumb. A study of factors influencing results in 1000 cases. J Bone Joint Surg Am 1971;53(7):1332–42.

range of motion. The patient is educated on the signs of infection and silicone-induced synovitis. If the diagnosis is delayed, infection may spread to involve the silicone rod, which requires removal.[32]

After a period of at least 3 months, the patient is returned to the operating room for the second stage. In the interim, the silicone rod has served as a gliding prosthesis around which a new pulley system has formed. All the advantages of using wide awake anesthesia for flexor tendon repairs, such as reduction gapping, avoidance of bunching, triggering, maximizing sheath preservation, and facilitating patient education, also apply in 2-stage tendon repairs.[7]

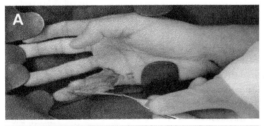
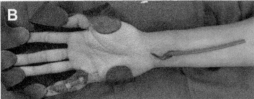
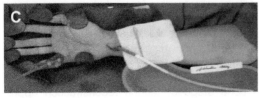

Fig. 1. (*A–C*) Stage 1 of 2-stage tendon reconstruction, (*A*) first preserving the distal flexor remnants. (*B*) The authors reconstruct the pulleys and (*C*) pull through the silicone rod.

Unlike the first stage, the second stage is performed using the wide awake technique. The tendon graft is chosen and harvested. Potential sites of tendon graft harvest are palmaris longus, plantaris, extensor digitorum longus, flexor digitorum superficialis, extensor indicis proprius, and extensor digiti minimi. As noted above, if long grafts or multiple grafts are needed, the lower extremity is an option.[33] The extensor digitorum longus to the second, third, and fourth toes can be harvested, with a potential length of 30 cm.[33]

The proximal end of the silicone rod is sutured to the tendon graft and pulled through the reconstructed pulley system. Distally, the tendon is sutured over a button, and its integrity is tested (Video 4). The proximal end is tensioned provisionally and Pulvertaft weaves are performed to a functioning digital flexor: either the original muscle or a nearby finger flexor in end-to-side fashion. Wide awake anesthesia allows evaluation of which muscles have retained strength of flexion. Appropriate tensioning is crucial for good clinical outcome, and tension is adjusted first passively by restoring the natural cascade of the fingers. As the patient actively flexes and extends, the Pulvertaft weave can be either tightened or loosened to achieve the ability to fully flex and extend. The optimal final result is full active extension and full flexion into the palm (Video 5).

The hand is placed into a dorsal blocking splint with the wrist in 30° of flexion, the metacarpophalangeal joints in 90° of flexion, and the interphalangeal joints in full extension.[34] Close postoperative follow-up and adherence to hand therapy protocols are essential for good outcomes. Passive place and hold may lead to tendon bunching rather than gliding within the pulley system.[35] The strength of the tendon-tendon interface was already tested intraoperatively, which gives the surgeon greater confidence in the repairs during early active motion.

Complications, such as tendon gapping, bowstringing, tendon rupture, residual tendon, or scar, causing a lumbrical plus deformity or quadrigia, which are difficult to determine without active flexion from the patient, can be minimized with wide awake anesthesia. Gapping may occur in 7% of patients after tendon repair.[7] With active pull-through, gapping can be determined and addressed during time of surgery.[36–38] Bowstringing can be seen with active motion, and the pulleys can then be reconstructed.

In the event of tendon rupture, reexploration is indicated before the pulleys have the chance to scar. Triggering may occur as the bulky tendon repair catches on pulleys and is best prevented by identifying the problem intraoperatively and addressing it by reducing tendon bulk or excising

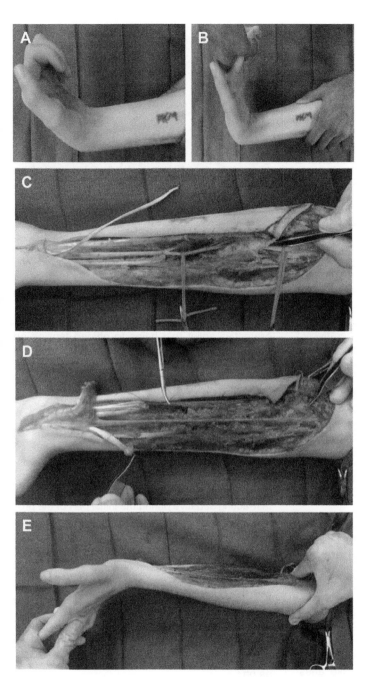

Fig. 2. (*A*, *B*) In this patient with Volkmann contracture, (*C*) the authors start with contracture release and perform neurolysis. (*D*) Next, the muscles and tendons are released, (*E*) with a new and improved Volkmann angle.

portion of the pulley. Despite these measures, triggering may still occur during the postoperative period. If there is no improvement with a trial of hand therapy, reexploration and release of trigger points are indicated. Partial tendon laceration may be a cause of triggering as well, which can be addressed by either trimming the tendon or venting the tethering pulley.

Quadrigia occurs when one of the FDP tendons to the ulnar 3 digits are shortened. Because these 3 tendons share a common muscle belly, if the

flexion of one of the tendons is restricted, the muscle cannot fully contract and rest of the finger cannot flex completely. Quadrigia results in inability to make a full fist or weakened grip. This condition is best diagnosed intraoperatively with wide awake anesthesia with the patient actively flexing.

The lumbrical plus deformity occurs when the interphalangeal joints paradoxically extend with active flexion. The lumbricals originate from the FDP and are relaxed when the FDP and FDS are contracting. If the FDP is transected at a point distal to the lumbrical origin, the force exerted does not translate to flexing the finger; instead the force is transmitted to the extensor mechanism. The lumbrical plus deformity may also occur if the tendon graft is too long, in which case during wide awake surgery, the problem can be identified as the patient actively flexes. The deformity can be corrected intraoperatively by adjusting the tension on the flexor tendon graft, or if necessary, by releasing the lumbrical muscle. Wide awake anesthesia is a powerful tool to prevent the lumbrical-plus deformity.

Tendon Transfers

One of the major challenges of tendon transfers is the determination of appropriate tensioning. An awake patient's active pull-through helps to determine the appropriate tension.[9] The integrity of the Pulvertaft weave is also tested to confirm adequate strength. Interestingly, cortical adaption after tendon transfer may occur quickly as the patient is asked to test the transfer intraoperatively.[8]

For primary tendon transfers, the tendons of interest are exposed and dissected free while under 20 minutes of tourniquet time. In the patient shown in Video 6, an extensor lag was identified when the patient was asked to actively extend his index finger. Index to long finger end-to-side transfer was performed using a Pulvertaft weave. The tendon transfer was provisionally sutured. Then, the tourniquet was deflated, and the patient actively flexed and extended the fingers. Accurate tensioning under wide awake anesthesia allowed full extension (Video 7).

Wide awake anesthesia can be useful even in situations of complex tendon transfers that require large areas of dissection. In this case example, the patient has fixed flexion at the wrist and fingers with inability to actively flex from a Volkmann contracture (**Fig. 2**A). In the first operation, the contracture was released, and neurolysis was performed under general anesthesia (**Fig. 2**). The Volkmann angle is much improved as result. The second stage for tendon transfers to re-create active finger flexion was performed under wide awake anesthesia. After tenolysing the flexor tendons to ensure good excursion of the tendons (Video 8), Extensor carpi radialis longus (ECRL) to FDP and brachioradialis to EDC tendon transfers were performed (**Fig. 3**). The sedation was discontinued, and the patient was asked to actively flex to demonstrate return of finger flexion (Video 9). Possible areas of triggering were checked to ensure the patient could fully flex while also being able to extend the fingers.

Intraoperative patient participation also serves an educational purpose as the patient is taught how to perform active motion immediately to ensure

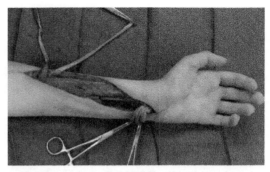

Fig. 3. The authors dissected out the planned tendon transfers: ECRL to FDP and brachioradialis to FPL.

understanding of the new pull vectors (Video 10). Intraoperative patient education is especially important during tendon transfers. Using the opportunity during the time of surgery to educate the patient on how to work their new tendon transfers leads to a more informed and more satisfied patient.[8]

Postoperatively, the patient was placed into a protective splint that helps to offload tension on the tendon transfers. After a 4-week period of immobilization to allow healing of the tendon transfers, an active motion protocol is initiated.

SUMMARY

Wide awake local anesthesia is a very useful technique for secondary and complex tendon reconstruction and may minimize common complications associated with this challenging clinical problem. The approach is modified by using a fast-acting sedative during the initial part of the procedure with a tourniquet for the first 20 minutes. The patient is awakened during the critical portion to evaluate the strength, gliding ability, and range of motion of the tendon reconstruction. In the authors' experience, it balances optimizing patient comfort with benefits of active patient motion.

SUPPLEMENTARY DATA

Supplementary data related to this article can be found online at https://doi.org/10.1016/j.hcl.2018.08.004.

REFERENCES

1. Beredjiklian PK. Biologic aspects of flexor tendon laceration and repair. J Bone Joint Surg Am 2003; 85:539–50.
2. Momeni A, Grauel E, Chang J. Complications after flexor tendon injuries. Hand Clin 2010;26:179–89.
3. Elliot D, Moiemen NS, Flemming AF, et al. The rupture rate of acute flexor tendon repairs mobilized by the controlled active motion regimen. J Hand Surg Br 1994;19:607–12.

4. Taras JS, Gray RM, Culp RW. Complications of flexor tendon injuries. Hand Clin 1994;10:93–109.
5. Nelson R, Higgins A, Conrad J, et al. The wide-awake approach to dupuytren's disease: fasciectomy under local anesthetic with epinephrine. Hand (N Y) 2010;5:117–24.
6. Lalonde DH, Kozin S. Tendon disorders of the hand. Plast Reconstr Surg 2011;128:1e–14e.
7. Higgins A, Lalonde DH, Bell M, et al. Avoiding flexor tendon repair rupture with intraoperative total active movement examination. Plast Reconstr Surg 2010; 126:941–5.
8. Bezuhly M, Sparkes GL, Higgins A, et al. Immediate thumb extension following extensor indicis proprius-to-extensor pollicis longus tendon transfer using the wide-awake approach. Plast Reconstr Surg 2007;119: 1507–12.
9. Lalonde DH. Wide-awake extensor indicis proprius to extensor pollicis longus tendon transfer. J Hand Surg Am 2014;39:2297–9.
10. Mackley CL, Marks JG Jr, Anderson BE. Delayed-type hypersensitivity to lidocaine. Arch Dermatol 2003;139:343–6.
11. Carazo JL, Morera BS, Colom LP, et al. Allergic contact dermatitis from ethyl chloride and benzocaine. Dermatitis 2009;20:E13–5.
12. Kennedy KS, Cave RH. Anaphylactic reaction to lidocaine. Arch Otolaryngol Head Neck Surg 1986; 112:671–3.
13. Lalonde D, Martin A. Tumescent local anesthesia for hand surgery: improved results, cost effectiveness, and wide-awake patient satisfaction. Arch Plast Surg 2014;41:312–6.
14. Prasetyono TO. Tourniquet-free hand surgery using the one-per-mil tumescent technique. Arch Plast Surg 2013;40:129–33.
15. Lalonde D, Eaton C, Amadio P, et al. Wide-awake hand and wrist surgery: a new horizon in outpatient surgery. Instr Course Lect 2015;64:249–59.
16. McKee DE, Lalonde DH, Thoma A, et al. Optimal time delay between epinephrine injection and incision to minimize bleeding. Plast Reconstr Surg 2013;131:811–4.
17. Lalonde D, Bell M, Benoit P, et al. A multicenter prospective study of 3,110 consecutive cases of elective epinephrine use in the fingers and hand: the Dalhousie Project clinical phase. J Hand Surg Am 2005;30:1061–7.
18. Zhang JX, Gray J, Lalonde DH, et al. Digital necrosis after lidocaine and epinephrine injection in the flexor tendon sheath without phentolamine rescue. J Hand Surg Am 2017;42:e119–23.
19. Ruiter T, Harter T, Miladore N, et al. Finger amputation after injection with lidocaine and epinephrine. Eplasty 2014;14:ic43.
20. Rosenbloom AL. Limitation of finger joint mobility in diabetes mellitus. J Diabet Complications 1989;3: 77–87.
21. Yang G, McGlinn EP, Chung KC. Management of the stiff finger: evidence and outcomes. Clin Plast Surg 2014;41:501–12.
22. Jupiter JB, Pess GM, Bour CJ. Results of flexor tendon tenolysis after replantation in the hand. J Hand Surg Am 1989;14:35–44.
23. Diao E, Eaton RG. Total collateral ligament excision for contractures of the proximal interphalangeal joint. J Hand Surg Am 1993;18:395–402.
24. Mohler LR, Pedowitz RA, Lopez MA, et al. Effects of tourniquet compression on neuromuscular function. Clin Orthop Relat Res 1999;359:213–20.
25. Concannon MJ, Kester CG, Welsh CF, et al. Patterns of free-radical production after tourniquet ischemia: implications for the hand surgeon. Plast Reconstr Surg 1992;89:846–52.
26. Tang JB. Wide-awake primary flexor tendon repair, tenolysis, and tendon transfer. Clin Orthop Surg 2015;7:275–81.
27. Boyes JH, Stark HH. Flexor-tendon grafts in the fingers and thumb. A study of factors influencing results in 1000 cases. J Bone Joint Surg Am 1971;53:1332–42.
28. Brug E, Stedtfeld HW. Results of 2-stage flexor tendon transplantation on zone 2. Handchirurgie 1979;11:127–30 [in German].
29. Wehbe MA, Mawr B, Hunter JM, et al. Two-stage flexor-tendon reconstruction. Ten-year experience. J Bone Joint Surg Am 1986;68:752–63.
30. Chong JK, Cramer LM, Culf NK. Combined two-stage tenoplasty with silicone rods for multiple flexor tendon injuries in "no-man's-land". J Trauma 1972;12:104–21.
31. Hume EL, Hutchinson DT, Jaeger SA, et al. Biomechanics of pulley reconstruction. J Hand Surg Am 1991;16:722–30.
32. Amadio PC, Wood MB, Cooney WP 3rd, et al. Staged flexor tendon reconstruction in the fingers and hand. J Hand Surg Am 1988;13:559–62.
33. Hunter JM, Salisbury RE. Flexor-tendon reconstruction in severely damaged hands. A two-stage procedure using a silicone-dacron reinforced gliding prosthesis prior to tendon grafting. J Bone Joint Surg Am 1971;53:829–58.
34. Farnebo S, Chang J. Practical management of tendon disorders in the hand. Plast Reconstr Surg 2013;132:841e–53e.
35. Higgins A, Lalonde DH. Flexor tendon repair postoperative rehabilitation: the Saint John protocol. Plast Reconstr Surg Glob Open 2016;4:e1134.
36. Tang JB, Zhou X, Pan ZJ, et al. Strong digital flexor tendon repair, extension-flexion test, and early active flexion: experience in 300 tendons. Hand Clin 2017;33:455–63.
37. Lalonde DH. Conceptual origins, current practice, and views of wide awake hand surgery. J Hand Surg Eur Vol 2017;42:886–95.
38. Lalonde D, Higgins A. Wide awake flexor tendon repair in the finger. Plast Reconstr Surg Glob Open 2016;4:e797.

Practice in Wide-Awake Hand Surgery
Differences Between United Kingdom and Cyprus

Constantinos Kritiotis, MD, EBHS[a,b,*], Alistair Phillips, FRCS[c],
Lindsay Muir, MB, MChOrth, FRCS (Orth)[a,d],
Zafar Naqui, MBBS, FRCS (Orth)[a,d]

KEYWORDS

- Wide-awake surgery • Local anesthesia • Lidocaine • Adrenaline • Hand surgery • Tourniquet
- WALANT

KEY POINTS

- Cyprus is a country without universal health care coverage, whereas in the United Kingdom, the presence of the National Health Service (NHS) guarantees universal health care coverage for the entire population.
- In Cyprus, wide-awake local anesthetic no tourniquet (WALANT) is gaining in popularity among patients because of its financial savings as well as the fact that patients do not want to receive a general anesthetic for their procedure.
- In the United Kingdom, WALANT procedures can be done without preoperative checks and tests; therefore, patients can have their procedure in shorter time than patients who are going to have any other method of anesthesia.
- In both countries, the use of WALANT leads to high patient satisfaction and optimum results, especially for dynamic procedures.

INTRODUCTION

Cyprus is an island country of 800,000 people in the Eastern Mediterranean. There is a significant influx of tourists in the summer months, with the tourist industry the cornerstone of the local economy. There is no universal health care covering the entire population of the island, with 20% of the population having no free access to public hospitals. Therefore, a significant percentage of the population prefers to attend private hospitals, which are paid either by private health insurance companies or by the patients themselves with self-pay care. A clear majority of patients attending private hospitals are self-paying patients who pay for their own treatment.

The United Kingdom has a diverse population of approximately 65 million inhabitants. Since 1948 it has had universal health care with the National Health Service (NHS). Every member of the public has free access to primary health care providers, such as general practitioners and hospitals emergency departments, as well as tertiary hospitals and specialists. There are also private hospitals

Disclosure: No financial interest or funding has been received for the completion of this article.
[a] Manchester Hand Centre, Salford Royal NHS Foundation Trust, Manchester, UK; [b] Iasis Private Hospital, 8 Voriou Ipirou Street, Paphos 8036, Cyprus; [c] Orthopaedic Department, University Hospital Southampton NHS Foundation Trust, Southampton General Hospital, Mailpoint 45, Tremona Road, Southampton SO16 6YD, UK; [d] Orthopaedic Department, Salford Royal Hospital, Stott Lane, Salford M6 8HD, UK
* Corresponding author. Iasis Private Hospital, 8 Voriou Ipirou Street, Paphos 8036, Cyprus.
E-mail address: Kritiotis@gmail.com

Hand Clin 35 (2019) 43–50
https://doi.org/10.1016/j.hcl.2018.08.007

that patients can access on a self-paying basis or through their private insurance providers.

DIFFERENCES IN ACCESS TO HAND SURGEONS IN THE TWO COUNTRIES

In Cyprus, patients are self-referred to specialist care. As such, patients who believe they have a hand problem seek a hand specialist opinion, bypassing general practitioners and other primary health care providers. In the United Kingdom, patients who go through the NHS have to be referred to a hand surgeon by a general practitioner or by the emergency department of a hospital. In both countries, the patients have a consultation with a hand surgeon and are offered the appropriate treatment, either surgical or nonsurgical. If patients need to have a surgical procedure, they discuss the procedure and the options of required anesthesia with their surgeon.

Patients who opt to have their procedures wide awake do not attend preoperative tests because local anesthesia procedures are considered extremely safe.[1–5] On the contrary, patients who undergo sedation, general anesthesia, or regional anesthesia must go through preoperative tests. In the authors' hospital in Manchester, England, the mean waiting time to go through preoperative testing is 1 month to 2 months. The waiting time for any hand surgical procedure is approximately a month.

In Cyprus, in the private health care hospital where the lead author (CK) works, preoperative tests can be done on the date of the consultation if the patient chooses sedation with an anesthesiologist. Anesthesiologist services and testing, however, can add a significant financial burden to the patient. There is no waiting time or testing for elective hand surgical procedures that are performed wide awake.

ACCEPTABILITY OF WIDE-AWAKE LOCAL ANESTHESIA PROCEDURES

Most patients are scared of the prospect of having their procedures done under local anesthesia because they are afraid that they might feel pain. They are also afraid that once a procedure starts there will be no way out. One of the main factors for patients in Cyprus to accept having their procedures wide awake is the significant cost savings because most patients are self-paying patients. Additionally, the fact that few anesthetists in Cyprus can perform regional blocks means that many patients must have general anesthesia to have hand surgery. This involves extensive preoperative tests as well as hospitalization.

In the United Kingdom, where patients pay nothing regardless of the method of anesthesia used (wide-awake, regional block, or general anesthesia), then it is up to the clinician to highlight the clinical benefits, safety, and efficiency of the WALANT method. Because patients do not need to go through preoperative testing and medical consultations, then they can have their procedure on short notice. Furthermore, if the clinical advantages of wide-awake local anesthesia are explained to patients, they are more likely to consent to it. A comparison of the patient experience on the day of a WALANT hand surgical procedure in the NHS in the United Kingdom versus in Cyprus is shown in **Fig. 1**.

DIFFERENCES IN LOCAL ANESTHESIA FOR WIDE-AWAKE HAND SURGERY IN THE TWO COUNTRIES

In Cyprus, the authors use 20 mL of lidocaine 2% and 1 mL of adrenaline 1:1000, diluted in 100 mL of normal saline. This creates a mixture of 0.33% lidocaine with 1:120,000 adrenaline, which ths authors have found efficient and effective for the procedures.

In Manchester, the authors either use a 10 mL of lidocaine, 1% ampule in which 1 mL of adrenaline 1:10,000 is added. For bigger procedures, a 100-mL bag of normal saline, out of which 40 mL of normal saline is removed, and then 1 mL of adrenaline 1:1000 to 20 mL of lidocaine 1% and 20 mL of levobupivacaine 5 mg/mL are added.

In Salford Royal NHS Foundation Trust in the UK, the authors have access to a former theatre storage room, which has been converted into a non-clean air theatre called the injection center. This is used for x-ray–guided injections and small day cases. Until recently it has been used for carpal tunnel decompressions and trigger finger releases. Recently the authors have started to convert the cases done there to WALANT cases that do not need metalwork (trapeziectomies, tendon transfers, Dupuytren releases, and so forth). This is usually staffed by 4 theatre staff (2 scrub nurses, 1 runner, and 1 operating department practitioner who acts as an anesthetic nurse). Theatre turnaround is approximately 20 minutes and the injection is carried out either in the ward or in recovery. Patients enter the theatre in theatre gowns.

In Paphos, Cyprus, patients are injected in the office and then taken to the theatre in their normal clothes. A gown is placed on top along with theatre cap and shoe covers, and patients enter the theatre in this way. The theatre staff is composed of a scrub nurse and a runner. No anesthetic nurse is used. In **Table 1**, similarities and differences

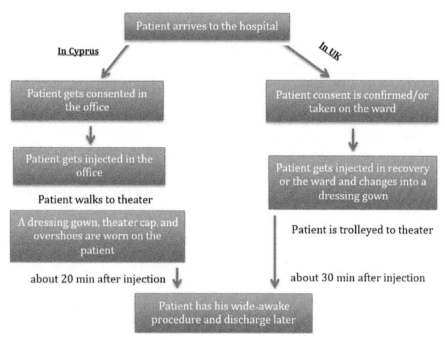

Fig. 1. A comparison of the patient experience on the day of a WALANT hand surgical procedure in the NHS in the UK and in Cyprus.

between the 2 countries regarding theatre setup are highlighted. Postoperatively, the patient attends outpatient appointments and hand therapy sessions as scheduled.

The authors used a questionnaire in both countries to assess the patients' perspectives as well as satisfaction with the use of WALANT. The questionnaire for the use of WALANT in the United Kingdom was carried out retrospectively (telephone questionnaire) and it included the questions that are in **Box 1**. The results were calculated on a visual analog scale score from 1 to 10, with 1 the least and 10 the most. The questionnaire for the use of WALANT in Cyprus was carried out on the day of surgery and it included preoperative as well as postoperative questions.

Table 1
Comparison of theatre setup in the United Kingdom and in Cyprus

Theatre Setup	United Kingdom (Manchester)	Cyprus (Paphos)
Surgical team	Surgeon and assistant (trainee)	Surgeon (scrub nurse assists)
Theatre staff	4 (2 scrub nurses, 1 operating department practitioner, and 1 runner)	2 (1 scrub nurse and 1 runner)
Theatre space	Any (can be nonclean air theatre)	Any (can be nonclean air theatre)
Surgical sets	Disposable (depending on case)	Standard
Monitoring	Sometimes	Not usually
Turnover time	Approximately 20 min	Approximately 20 min
Local anaesthetic injection taking place in	Recovery/ward	Office
Patient attire	Theatre gown	Standard clothes with gown on top
Antiseptic used	Chlorhexidine	Chlorhexidine
Discharge	From ward after 30 min	Straight from theatre

Box 1
Wide-awake local anesthetic no tourniquet telephone questionnaire performed in the United Kingdom

1. How painful were the injections?
2. How painful was your procedure?
3. How afraid were you before the procedure knowing that it will be done under local anesthesia?
4. Would you have future procedures with this kind of anesthesia?
5. What were the reason you had your procedure wide awake?
    a. Afraid of general anesthesia
    b. Surgeon mentioned better results
    c. Surgeon mentioned safety
    d. I was not offered another method
    e. Other

The results were calculated on a visual analog scale from 1 to 10, with 1 the least and 10 the

Box 2
Questionnaire for wide-awake local anesthetic no tourniquet used in Cyprus

Preoperative questions

What scares you the most for having your procedure wide awake?

Did you have any other procedures under local anesthesia (yes/no)?

How painful were the other procedures that you had under local anesthesia (1–10)?

What was the reason for having your procedure wide awake?

- Did not want to stay in hospital
- Did not want general anesthesia
- Financial concern

Postoperative questions

How painful was the local anesthesia administration (1–10)?

How painful was your procedure (1–10)?

Did you have a top-up of your local anesthesia?

How comfortable were during your procedure (1–10)?

What was the biggest problem you faced during the procedure?

Would you do such a procedure wide awake again (yes/no)?

most. Some multiple-choice questions were added as well (**Box 2**).

Regarding the calculation of the financial benefits of WALANT in Cyprus, the authors used the information from the finance department of the private hospital where the lead author works. Specifically, the charges for a procedure that can be done either under WALANT versus general anesthesia (trapeziectomy) were compared.

In the United Kingdom, the collection of these data was slightly more complicated. The authors managed to clarify, however, that an NHS trust is paid the same tariff for a procedure irrespective of the anesthesia method used.

THE AUTHORS' CLINICAL DATA AND RESULTS

Table 2 presents a summary of the authors' cases done in Salford Royal NHS Foundation Trust and Trafford General Hospital on behalf of the Manchester Hand Centre from July 2017 to March 2018 and the cases in Cyprus. One author (CK) did all the cases in both countries, either as head surgeon or assistant surgeon. The collection of this information was carried out through patient records (see **Table 2**). Of these patients, 2 required readmission in the hospital and wound débridement. The other complications were managed on an outpatient basis. Only 2 patients in Cyprus required anesthetic intervention. In the United Kingdom, of the 46 patients contacted, 33 agreed to answer the questionnaire in a telephone interview.

In Cyprus, the patients who had carpal tunnel decompressions as well as trigger finger releases were provided with this questionnaire and their responses included. The results are summarized in **Table 3**.

Regarding cost savings, the authors calculated the cost of a common hand surgery procedure (trapeziectomy) done under WALANT and under general anesthesia. **Table 4** presents a comparison of the hospital fees for a WALANT and general anesthesia for a trapeziectomy in Cyprus. The cost is in euros and excludes the surgeon fees. **Table 5** shows procedural costs in the NHS.

There is a strong financial incentive to implement WALANT in hospitals either in Cyprus or the United Kingdom. In Cyprus, the authors have shown that surgery costs can drop by 75%. These are savings directly benefiting the patients or their insurance companies. In the United Kingdom, the use of nonclean air theatres, the absence of an anesthetist, and the alleviation of the need for preoperative checks can lead both to significant cost cutting for the NHS and shortening of the waiting time for surgery (the wait for preoperative checks in the authors' hospital is approximately 6 weeks).

Table 2
Highlight of procedures performed under wide-awake local anesthetic no tourniquet

Procedures	Number Performed in Manchester	Number Performed in Cyprus	Remarks and Complications
Open reduction internal fixation of metacarpals and phalanges	11	8	
Trapeziectomy and tendon suspension	5	9	1 superficial infection (UK) 1 CRPS (Cyprus)
Collateral ligament repair with bone anchor	3	5	
Flexor tendon surgery (repair, tenolysis, first-stage flexor reconstruction)	4	10	Hematoma due to poor coagulation control One infection in Cyprus due to poor patient compliance
Removal of metal from hand and tenolysis	12	0	
Centralization of extensor tendon in the hand	3	0	
Dupuytren contracture fasciectomy (limited or needle)	4	7	
EIP to EPL transfer	3	0	Excellent outcome to all
FCR to EDC transfer	3	0	One deep infection, excellent functional outcome
Joint fusions (metacarpophalangeal, proximal interphalangeal, or carpometacarpal joints) using screw or locking plate	4	0	Union achieved in all (1 was revision)
ECU débridement and sheath reconstruction using extensor retinaculum flap	1	1	
Excision of ulnar head with extensor tendon buddying	1	0	Patient required light sedation but no analgesia. Able to cooperate during transfer

Abbreviations: CRPS, Complex Regional Pain Syndrome; ECU, Extensor Carpi Ulnaris; EDC, Extensor Digitorum Communis; EIP, Extensor Indicis Proprius; EPL, Extensor Pollicis Longus; FCR, Flexor Carpi Radialis

As far as the patient perspective about WALANT is concerned, patients in both countries are concerned by the prospect of having their procedures under WALANT at approximately 45% in both countries. Patient education and an honest consultation can help improve these concerns. Also, as surgeons become more familiar with the technique, they can offer it to more suitable candidates, emphasizing that the conversion rate of WALANT to general anesthesia is very small, less than 1% in Cyprus and none so far in the United Kingdom.

Cost cutting is one of the reasons that 18% of the authors' Cypriot patients chose WALANT, something that is not applicable in United Kingdom patients because of the universal health care coverage. The implementation of WALANT lists and the introduction of WALANT acute clinics for routine hand trauma in the United Kingdom, however, can significantly cut the costs of day surgery cases. This is the route by which a clear majority of hand surgery cases are performed.

Table 3
Comparison of outcomes of WALANT between the United Kingdom and Cyprus

Questions	United Kingdom (Average Scores or Results)	Cyprus (Average Score or Results)
How painful were the injections?	4.6/10	3.7/10
How painful was your procedure?	2.3/10	1,6/10
How afraid were you before the procedure knowing that it will be done under local anesthesia?	5/10	4.6/10
Would you have future procedures with this kind of anesthesia?	31/33: Yes 2/33: No	144/145: Yes 1/145: No
What was the reason for having this procedure under wide awake?	a. Afraid of general anesthesia: 1 b. Surgeon mentioned better results: 11 c. Surgeon mentioned safety: 13 d. I was not offered another method: 5 e. Other: 2 (1 had water before surgery and 1 specifically requested local anesthesia)	a. Not wanting hospital stay: 46% b. Afraid of general anesthesia: 36% c. Cost savings: 18%

Regarding the authors' injection technique, approximately half of the authors' patients in the United Kingdom experience pain during the injection. Improvements can be implemented to reduce this number, such as the addition of sodium bicarbonate to the local anesthetic to increase the pH and the introduction of smaller needles (see Margie Wheelock and colleagues' article, "The Canadian Model for Instituting Wide Awake Hand Surgery in Our Hospitals," in this issue, for new ways to decrease the pain of injection).

In short, the authors have achieved excellent safety, cost, and patient satisfaction rates in both countries and have shown that WALANT is transferable between 2 very different health systems. LeBlanc and colleagues[6] have shown that WALANT can be twice as efficient and for a quarter of the cost for small hand surgery procedures. The indications are expanding greatly. WALANT has been used for many procedures from small cases[6–12] and increasingly for larger cases. The benefits of intraoperative active movements testing of surgical repairs are proving clinically effective in flexor tendon repairs,[13–20] lacertus release,[21,22] wrist arthroscopy,[23] trapeziectomy,[24,25] and digital revasularization.[26]

The other benefits of WALANT, discussed previously, are all transferable between health care systems, whether privately or state funded. With the cost of health care rising due to ever more expensive implants, salaries, indemnity, and litigation, WALANT brings a truly win (patient), win (surgeon), win (bill payer–insurer/self-funder), and win (health care provider) situation. Increasingly state-funded health systems, such as the NHS, struggle to meet the demand for surgical services. A report released in September 2017 by Private Healthcare UK (www.privatehealth.co.uk) showed that the annual growth of patients paying for their treatment (self-funders) in the United Kingdom is between 15% and 25%. Offering WALANT as an

Table 4
Average cost comparison of Cyprus for use of WALANT versus other methods of anesthesia (surgeon fees excluded) per operation

Fees	WALANT	Other Methods of Anesthesia
Preoperative checks	0	107.5
Anesthetist fees	0	250
Theatre charges	250	250
Intravenous medication	0	195
Intravenous fluids	0	18
Giving sets	0	8
Day case bed	0	190
Total	250 euros	1018.50 euros

Table 5
Cost savings in the United Kingdom

Fees	WALANT	Other Method of Anesthesia
Preoperative checks	0 (not needed)	Up to 6 wk waiting time
Anesthetist fees	0	Same fees as surgeon
Theatre charges	Can be done in nonclean air theatres (procedures not requiring implants)	Needs clean air
Intravenous medication	0	Needed
Intravenous fluids	0	Needed in general anesthesia cases
Giving sets	0	Needed
Day case bed	Needed from before the procedure up to 30 min after conclusion of procedure	Can be converted to inpatient if patient has general anesthesia toward the end of the day
Tariff paid	Same regardless of anesthesia method	

alternative to traditional, more expensive alternatives may be one way that WALANT establishes itself as a routine standard of care. From there, only time and research will show if it should be the gold standard of care.

SUMMARY

There are many differences in the health care systems in the 2 countries. The NHS in the United Kingdom provides universal health care coverage, whereas Cyprus does not. By implementing WALANT in Cyprus, the authors have cut the costs of the service provided by at least 40% (in some cases this equals with cost savings of more than 1000 euros). In the United Kingdom, the omission of preoperative checks as well as the implementation of WALANT-only lists, without the presence of an anesthetist, can reduce both the cost and the mean waiting time for patients to have his procedure. The authors do not find their complication rate higher than with the use of other anesthesia methods, rendering WALANT a safe anesthesia method for hand surgery procedures. Finally, if patients are well educated prior to their procedures and told what to expect, they become active participants and are able to see in some instances the results of their procedure prior to exiting the operating room. This reassures them about the outcome, enhances the patient/surgeon relationship and trust, and increases their satisfaction.

REFERENCES

1. Jagodzinski NA, Ibish S, Furniss D. Surgical site infection after hand surgery outside the operating theatre: a systematic review. J Hand Surg Eur Vol 2017;42:289–94.

2. Lalonde D, Martin A. Tumescent local anesthesia for hand surgery: improved results, cost effectiveness, and wide-awake patient satisfaction. Arch Plast Surg 2014;41:312–6.

3. Davison PG, Cobb T, Lalonde DH. The patient's perspective on carpal tunnel surgery related to the type of anesthesia: a prospective cohort study. Hand (N Y) 2013;8:47–53.

4. Rhee PC, Fischer MM, Rhee LS, et al. Cost savings and patient experiences of a clinic-based, wide-awake hand surgery program at a military medical center: a critical analysis of the first 100 procedures. J Hand Surg Am 2017;42:e139–47.

5. Teo I, Lam W, Muthayya P, et al. Patients' perspective of wide-awake hand surgery–100 consecutive cases. J Hand Surg Eur Vol 2013;38:992–9.

6. Leblanc MR, Lalonde J, Lalonde DH. A detailed cost and efficiency analysis of performing carpal tunnel surgery in the main operating room versus the ambulatory setting in Canada. Hand (N Y) 2007;2: 173–8.

7. Barros MF, da Rocha Luz Júnior A, Roncaglio B, et al. Evaluation of surgical treatment of carpal tunnel syndrome using local anesthesia. Rev Bras Ortop 2016;51:36–9.

8. Codding JL, Bhat SB, Ilyas AM. An economic analysis of MAC versus WALANT: a trigger finger release surgery case study. Hand (N Y) 2017;12: 348–51.

9. Foster BD, Sivasundaram L, Heckmann N, et al. Surgical approach and anesthetic modality for carpal tunnel release: a nationwide database study with health care cost implications. Hand (N Y) 2017;12: 162–7.

10. Hustedt JW, Chung A, Bohl DD, et al. Comparison of postoperative complications associated with anesthetic choice for surgery of the hand. J Hand Surg Am 2017;42:1–8.e5.

11. Leblanc MR, Lalonde DH, Thoma A, et al. Is main operating room sterility really necessary in carpal tunnel surgery? A multicenter prospective study of minor procedure room field sterility surgery. Hand (N Y) 2011;6:60–3.

12. Nabhan A, Ishak B, Al-Khayat J, et al. Endoscopic carpal tunnel release using a modified application technique of local anesthesia: safety and effectiveness. J Brachial Plex Peripher Nerve Inj 2008;3:11.

13. Gibson PD, Sobol GL, Ahmed IH. Zone II flexor tendon repairs in the United States: trends in current management. J Hand Surg Am 2017;42:e99–108.

14. Higgins A, Lalonde DH, Bell M, et al. Avoiding flexor tendon repair rupture with intraoperative total active movement examination. Plast Reconstr Surg 2010; 126:941–5.

15. Lalonde DH. An evidence-based approach to flexor tendon laceration repair. Plast Reconstr Surg 2011; 127:885–90.

16. Lalonde DH, Kozin S. Tendon disorders of the hand. Plast Reconstr Surg 2011;128:1e–14e.

17. Lalonde DH, Martin AL. Wide-awake flexor tendon repair and early tendon mobilization in zones 1 and 2. Hand Clin 2013;29:207–13.

18. Lalonde DH. Decreasing tendon rupture and tenolysis with wide awake surgery. BMC Proc 2015;9:A66.

19. Tang JB, Zhou X, Pan ZJ, et al. Strong digital flexor tendon repair, extension-flexion test, and early active flexion: experience in 300 tendons. Hand Clin 2017;33:455–63.

20. Lalonde DH. Conceptual origins, current practice, and views of wide awake hand surgery. J Hand Surg Eur Vol 2017;42:886–95.

21. Hagert E. Clinical diagnosis and wide-awake surgical treatment of proximal median nerve entrapment at the elbow: a prospective study. Hand (N Y) 2013;8:41–6.

22. Lalonde DH. Lacertus syndrome: a commonly missed and misdiagnosed median nerve entrapment syndrome. BMC Proc 2015;9:A74.

23. Hagert E, Lalonde DH. Wide-awake wrist arthroscopy and open TFCC repair. J Wrist Surg 2012;1: 55–60.

24. Farhangkhoee H, Lalonde J, Lalonde DH. Wide-awake trapeziectomy: video detailing local anesthetic injection and surgery. Hand (N Y) 2011;6: 466–7.

25. Mckee D, Lalonde DH. Wide awake trapeziectomy for thumb basal joint arthritis. Plast Reconstr Surg Glob Open 2017;5:e1435.

26. Wong J, Lin CH, Chang NJ, et al. Digital revascularization and replantation using the wide-awake hand surgery technique. J Hand Surg Eur Vol 2017;42: 621–5.

Wide Awake Hand Surgery Under Local Anesthesia No Tourniquet in South America

Pedro José Pires Neto, MD[a],*, Samuel Ribak, MD, PhD[b],
Trajano Sardenberg, MD, PhD[c]

KEYWORDS

- Wide awake hand surgery • Epinephrine finger • Tourniquet-free • Local anesthesia
- Brazil hand surgery • Carpal tunnel bilateral • Ambulatory surgery • Arteriovenous fistulas

KEY POINTS

- Brazilian hand surgery groups located in Minas Gerais, Campinas, Botucatu, and Rio de Janeiro implement the wide awake hand surgery under local anesthesia no tourniquet (WALANT) technique described by Dr Lalonde.
- A premixed 1% lidocaine solution with 1:100,000 epinephrine is not yet available in Brazil. The authors, therefore, mix their own. They add 0.2 mL of epinephrine (1.0 mg/mL) with a 1-mL syringe, to 20 mL of 1% lidocaine.
- Brazil is a massive country with a great diversity in services of hand surgery, including its methods of payments and costs. The differences in the public and private systems add to that variability. Early WALANT has shown advantages in all these different scenarios.
- By applying fairness in surgeon reimbursement, Brazilian health plan insurers can help spread this technique, which decreases patient cost and improves patient safety and results of surgery.

INTRODUCTION

In Brazil, most of the hand surgery is performed by surgeons who specialize in orthopedics and traumatology, with or without additional specialization in hand surgery. Sterling Bunnell's[1] book, *Surgery of the Hand*, was used as the primary reference text in training centers in Brazil in the 1960s and 1970s. The Spanish version, published in 1967, was titled *BUNNELL–BOYES–Cirurgia de la Mano*.[2] It explicitly discussed local anesthesia. On page 137, it stated "Si se utiliza en um dedo no debe contener epinefrina," meaning, "If used in a finger, it should not contain epinephrine." The restriction of epinephrine for local anesthesia of the hand became dogma among Brazilian hand surgeons, as it was in much of the rest of the world.

Brazil is a massive country with a large diversity of conditions for practicing medicine. The introduction of wide awake hand surgery under local anesthesia no tourniquet (WALANT) began mainly in the states of Minas Gerais (Belo Horizonte City) and São Paulo (Campinas, Botucatu, and São Paulo City), Brazil.

THE START OF WIDE AWAKE HAND SURGERY IN BRAZIL

In 1991, the Brazilian Society of Plastic Surgery asked Dr Pedro José Pires Neto, in Belo Horizonte,

Disclosure Statement: The authors have no financial interest to declare in relation to the content of this article.
[a] Department of Orthopaedic and Hand Surgery, Felício Rocho Hospital, Av. do Contorno 9530, Belo Horizonte, Minas Gerais 30110-934, Brazil; [b] Pontifical Catholic University of Campinas (PUC-Campinas), Av. John Boyd Dunlop - Jardim Ipaussurama, Campinas, São Paulo 13034-685, Brazil; [c] Departament of Surgery and Orthopedics, Botucatu Medical School, São Paulo State University, UNESP, Av. Professor Mario Rubens Montenegro s/n, Botucatu, São Paulo 18 618-687, Brazil
* Corresponding author.
E-mail address: pires@felicoop.org.br

Hand Clin 35 (2019) 51–58
https://doi.org/10.1016/j.hcl.2018.08.005
0749-0712/19/© 2018 Elsevier Inc. All rights reserved.

MG to evaluate an article investigating the use of local anesthesia with epinephrine for chicken's feet with no record of tissue necrosis. The author of the study, Dr Cesar Arunatega, further demonstrated safety by injecting anesthesia with epinephrine into his own and his wife's hands. Even though the article was not published, Brazilian hand surgeons became aware of this story. This significant historical event contributed to ending the myth of the danger of injecting epinephrine in the hand in Brazil.

In 2010, Dr Sérgio A. M. da Gama, from the Pontifical Catholic University (PUC) of Campinas, reported to his peers that he had just participated in a course in Philadelphia, Pennsylvania, where a Canadian surgeon had presented a local anesthesia technique using epinephrine without a tourniquet for surgical procedures of the wrists, hands, and fingers. On that occasion, Dr Gama stated that several American hand surgeons had criticized the safety of using epinephrine in hand surgeries, particularly in the finger. The Canadian physician, Dr Lalonde, defended himself by presenting the results of a large clinical prospective study involving the use of this technique as a routine procedure at the Saint John Regional Hospital, Dalhousie University, and in 5 other Canadian cities.[3,4] Dr Gama's comments did not create great excitement among his peers at that time. Nevertheless, the idea remained in some surgeons' minds. In public hospitals in Brazil, there was a chronic lack of available operating time for elective procedures, because of the lack of nurses, anesthetists, and other problems.

In 2012, Dr Lalonde attended the 32nd Brazilian Congress of Hand Surgery in São Paulo, where he showed his studies and expertise of the technique called Wide Awake Hand Surgery with only local anesthesia and epinephrine, and without a tourniquet, sedation, or anesthetist. The Brazilian physicians had an intense debate on the risks and benefits of the technique. One of the main concerns was the risk of the medical-legal issues in the case of complications during the surgery without the presence of an anesthetist. By comparing hand surgery to procedures performed by dentists with local anesthesia and without an anesthetist, Dr Lalonde diminished the concerns of the Brazilian surgeons.

At the end of 2012, in the university hospital of the medical school of São Paulo State University-UNESP in Botucatu, 3 surgeons (Drs Denis Varanda, Andrea C. Cortopassi, and Trajano Sardenberg) decided to implement the technique described by Dr Lalonde after studying the scientific literature in detail. However, premixed 1% lidocaine with 1:100,000 epinephrine was not available in Brazil. Thus, after studies on drug dilution, the following process was established by the surgeons. At the time of surgery, they used a 1.0-mL syringe to mix 0.2 mL of 1.0 mg/mL epinephrine hemitartrate with 20 mL of 1% lidocaine. Sodium bicarbonate was not used to buffer acidic burning discomfort because the possibility of errors was increased on adding a second drug to the lidocaine.

At the beginning of 2013, surgeons from the University Hospitals of Botucatu (UNESP) and Dr Samuel Ribak, from the Pontifical Catholic University of Campinas, SP (PUC Campinas), began a prospective study to evaluate the complications directly related to the use of epinephrine for local anesthesia in hand surgery. Simultaneously, they began teaching this technique of anesthesia and surgery to residents of medicine, orthopedics, traumatology, and hand surgery at the UNESP and Campinas (PUC). The first procedures included carpal tunnel syndrome (CTS), trigger finger, de Quervain disease, and benign tumors. The first 40 patients underwent surgery without complications. The use of the technique was then extended to trauma cases, such as extensor tendon injuries. They reported 488 hand procedures using the WALANT technique.[5] No cases of digital infarction, tissue necrosis, surgery suspension, tourniquet use, or intraoperative anesthesia assistance were reported.

In 2014, Ronaldo Novais Jr and colleagues[6] published the first study in Brazil on local anesthesia with epinephrine for hand surgery. They reported 41 patients who underwent operation without complications. In 2016, Marco Barros and his colleagues[7] published the results of 16 patients with CTS with WALANT without complications. Both studies reinforced the belief in South America that WALANT is safe and effective.

In 2014, Dr Marco Barros of Valadares, Brazil visited Dr Lalonde in Canada and suggested a method to mix medications to obtain 1% lidocaine with a 1:100,000 epinephrine, because many countries do not have premixed local anesthetic solutions. Dr Lalonde published Dr Barros' suggestion in the first textbook of wide awake hand surgery.[8] Dr Mario Kuwae, of Santa Isabel, Brazil, was the first Brazilian hand surgeon to visit Dr Lalonde in Canada in 2013. Drs Renata Pedra, Wilson Huang, Rafael Saleme, Caio Pina came after 2014.

In 2017, Dr Lalonde spoke again at the 37th Brazilian Congress of Hand Surgery in Belo Horizonte, MG. The session was a 4-hour course with many hand surgeons in attendance. After Dr Lalonde's lectures, a round table discussion took place with several Brazilian hand surgeons, reporting their experiences with WALANT in their daily practice. The conclusion was that WALANT has attractive advantages across the great diversity of hand

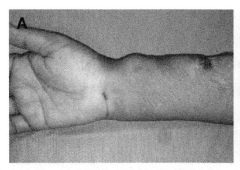
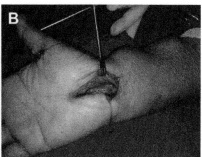

Fig. 1. (*A*) Blockade with lidocaine and epinephrine in carpal tunnel and trigger thumb release in a patient with arteriovenous fistula for hemodialysis. (*B*) Extended access for carpal tunnel release and synovectomy due to amyloidosis.

services, payment, and cost systems in both the public and the private sectors in Brazil. In 2017, Pedro Pires Neto and colleagues[9,10] published an article disseminating the WALANT technique to the orthopedic community.

THE APPLICATION OF WIDE AWAKE HAND SURGERY IN BRAZIL

Currently, half of the hand surgical procedures at the UNESP surgery center are performed under full sterility WALANT. The most common procedures are CTS, de Quervain disease, trigger finger, benign tumors, flexor and extensor tendon injuries, hand tendon transfers, and finger infections, which are similar to practices in other countries.[11] Surgeons there plan to initiate more frequent treatment of hand fractures, finger fusions, Dupuytren, and injuries to nerves and tendons of the wrist and forearm. They are also working on the creation of an operating room specifically designed to perform hand surgery with WALANT.

Surgeons from Botucatu have now used WALANT without a tourniquet, sedation, or an anesthetist in more than 2000 procedures with no complications related to epinephrine.

Dr Pedro Pires, while working at Felício Rocho Hospital in Belo Horizonte, MG, observed difficulties while performing tourniquet hand surgery in renal failure patients with arteriovenous fistulas for hemodialysis. Surgery without a tourniquet results in an increase in surgical time and blood loss. The introduction of the WALANT technique facilitated hand surgery by eliminating excessive bleeding and the tourniquet in these patients (**Fig. 1**). **Fig. 2** illustrates a WALANT trigger finger release in a patient with chronic renal failure and an arteriovenous fistula. WALANT also facilitates synovectomy in trigger finger and in carpal tunnel release in these patients. The synovectomy functions as a flexor tendon tenolysis in CTS. It is possible to observe isolated flexor tendons move

after synovectomy (**Fig. 3**). Renal insufficiency and amyloidosis cause a thickening and hardening of the epineurium, which lead to compression of the median nerve in the carpal tunnel. Debulking the nerve reduces the compression and improves its vascularity.[9]

The mastery and confidence acquired with WALANT in hemodialysis patients with arteriovenous fistulas stimulated hand surgeons in Belo Horizonte to perform other procedures. It has been particularly useful in cases where active motion during surgery allows for immediate evaluation of the results. WALANT enables intraoperative corrections. A good example is in the reduction of malrotated finger fractures after trauma. It is comforting to see convergent active finger movement toward the scaphoid tubercle before leaving the operating room (**Fig. 4**).

Functional results improve in tendon transfers because of the viewing of intraoperative active movement. The patient in **Fig. 5** suffered an injury to the extensors of the index finger, which was missed when the skin laceration was sutured.

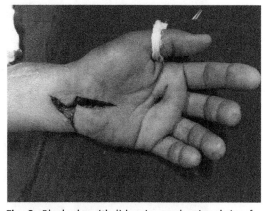

Fig. 2. Blockade with lidocaine and epinephrine for carpal tunnel release by extended access and trigger middle finger release in the member with arteriovenous fistula for hemodialysis.

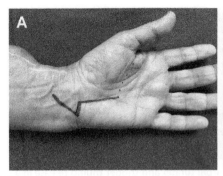
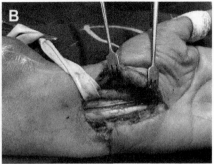

Fig. 3. (*A*) Blockade with lidocaine and epinephrine for carpal tunnel release by extended access in the member with arteriovenous fistula for hemodialysis. (*B*) Detail after synovectomy due to amyloidosis in patients with arteriovenous fistula for hemodialysis.

Two months later, the patient did not have active extension of the index finger. At that time, the distal tendon stump was sewn to the extensor tendon of the middle finger under WALANT. After the initial sutures, the ideal transfer tension was confirmed with patient active movement during the surgery. The WALANT technique facilitated his adherence to the rehabilitation program and improved the confidence of both the surgeon and the patient that a good result could be achieved.

Joint contractures and adhesions of tendons after phalangeal fractures are common after crushing injuries. There is a limitation that is often not severe but, depending on the patient's profession or sports participation, might be incapacitating. In **Fig. 6**, the patient needed full flexion to perform his professional activity. Tenolysis and capsulotomy

were performed with WALANT to improve the patient's function. To improve the patient's function, which allowed the patient to understand the degree of movement obtained during the surgery to help manage his expectations and motivate him during therapy.

Chronic injury to the sagittal band, which most commonly occurs in the middle finger on the radial side, allows the extensor tendon to dislocate to the interval between the third and fourth metacarpals heads. This condition can be disabling for patients. They sometimes require assistance from the opposite hand to open the hand normally. **Fig. 7** shows the sequence from the clinical diagnosis of the extensor apparatus dislocation to the final postoperative result. The investigators used a distally based central strip of the long finger extensor

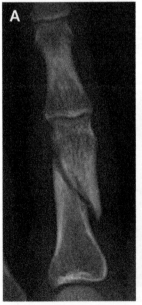
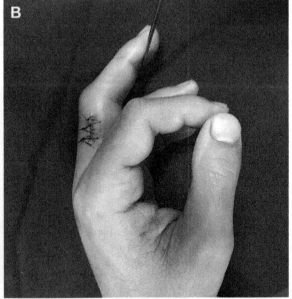

Fig. 4. (*A*) Radiography showing an oblique fracture with deviation at the proximal phalanx of the middle finger. (*B*) Miniaccess on the radial side of the proximal phalanx of the middle finger with pinning fixation. The finger actively moved during surgery to verify the stability of fixation with pins.

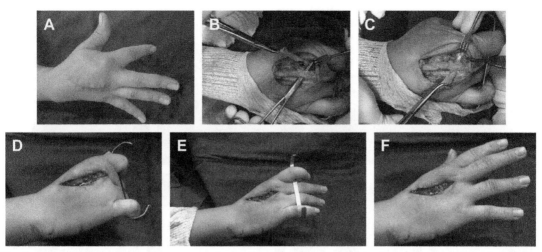

Fig. 5. Chronic injury of the extensor proprius and common tendons of the index finger. (*A*) The inability to actively extend the index finger. (*B, C*) The suturing of the extensor proprius of the index finger and common tendon of the middle finger using an end-to-side suture. (*D, E*) Active extension and flexion of the middle and ring fingers with index finger in protection. (*F*) Active extension of the fingers after suturing, showing level and symmetric tension among the fingers.

tendon to reconstruct the chronic injury of the sagittal band. The tendon strip went under the collateral ligament on the radial side of the metacarpophalangeal and was sutured back into the extensor apparatus. The intraoperative active movement enabled the adjustment of the tension to avoid undercorrection or overcorrection. In a condition whereby the deficiency is dynamic, it is ideal that the correction is also dynamic.

Recent research from PUC University from Campinas has prospectively compared median nerve release with bilateral CTS with and without WALANT in 106 patients who had surgery simultaneously or in 2 stages. Although not yet published, this study will present several advantages of WALANT, including a significant improvement of the Disabilities of Arm, Shoulder and Hand Questionnaire and a shorter time of return to work (**Fig. 8**).

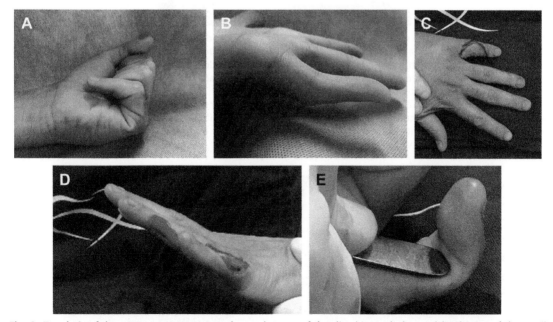

Fig. 6. Tenolysis of the extensor apparatus and capsulotomy of the distal interphalangeal (DIP) joint of the small finger. (*A, B*) Active movement of flexion and extension of the small finger showing limitations in flexion of the DIP and extension of the proximal interphalangeal. (*C*) The pinkie finger, after tenolysis of the extensor apparatus and dorsal DIP capsulotomy. (*D*) Active extension of the pinkie finger. (*E*) Detailed active flexion of the DIP joint.

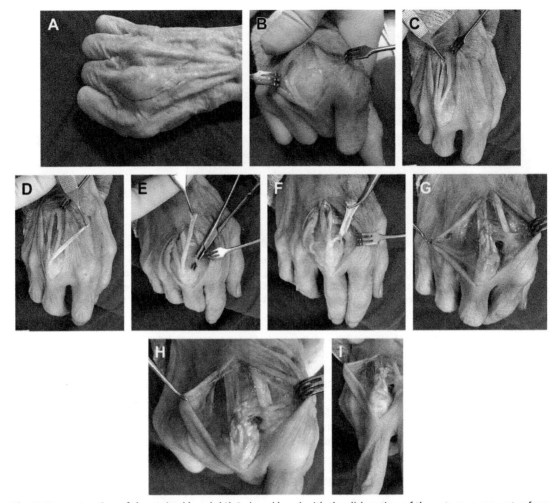

Fig. 7. Reconstruction of the sagittal band. (*A*) A closed hand with the dislocation of the extensor apparatus from the middle finger to the ulnar side of the third metacarpal head. (*B*) Dorsal access and visualization of the dislocated ulnar extensor apparatus owing to chronic injury of the radial side sagittal band. (*C*) The central strip of the extender apparatus is prepared. (*D*) Isolating the strip of the extensor apparatus. (*E*) Isolating the radial collateral ligament of the metacarpophalangeal of the middle finger through which the isolated central band of the extensor apparatus will be passed. (*F*) Passing the strip of the extensor apparatus under the radial side collateral ligament. (*G*) Suturing the strip in the extensor. (*H*) Testing the stability of the extensor apparatus on the third metacarpal head during active flexion. (*I*) Testing the stability of the extensor apparatus over the head of the third metacarpal during active extension.

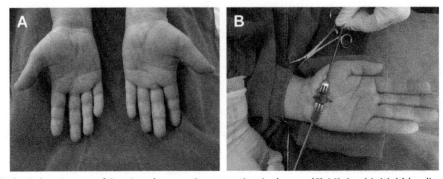

Fig. 8. (*A*) The ischemic area of 2 wrists that require operation is shown. (*B*) Minimal initial bleeding after skin incision.

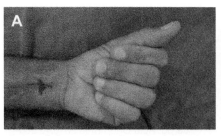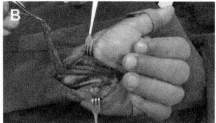

Fig. 9. (*A*) Trigger of the wrist, misdiagnosed as trigger in the third finger. (*B*) The tumor extending through the carpal tunnel during active flexion of the finger and showing intense synovitis. Smooth wrist and finger motion was confirmed during surgery after tumor removal.

The WALANT technique is very useful when the diagnosis is uncertain, such as in the case of a "trigger wrist," which was initially mistreated as trigger finger. In the patient in **Fig. 9**, the authors verified under WALANT that the triggering was caused by an angiomyolipoma in the carpal tunnel. The true cause became evident when the patient was asked to flex the finger intraoperatively.

Local flaps for fingertip coverage are an interesting indication for WALANT, as in the case illustrated in **Fig. 10**, where a thenar flap was performed. Active flexion of the finger was helpful to determine the proper location and dissection of

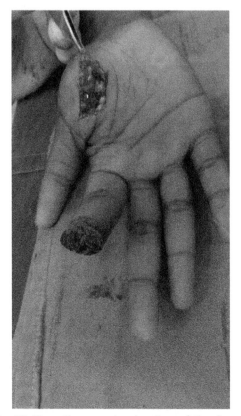

Fig. 10. Fingertip necrosis; elevation of the flap of adequate size.

the flap. Anesthesia was injected at 3 different points of the hand, and the epinephrine did not interfere with vascularization of the flap.

BRAZILIAN HEALTH CARE AND BENEFITS OF WIDE AWAKE HAND SURGERY UNDER LOCAL ANESTHESIA NO TOURNIQUET

In Brazil, there is a peculiar funding situation in the private system in which medical fees are defined by a patient's accommodation. If a patient is hospitalized in a private room, the insurer pays the surgeon his full fee for surgery. However, if a patient is hospitalized in a multipatient room, or if the procedure is performed on an outpatient basis, the surgeon is only funded at 50% of the fee. This situation has been a major obstacle to the increased use of the WALANT technique and has led to a waste of precious resources. Brazilian health plan insurers need to reap the rewards of decreased cost with increased patient safety and satisfaction, but without reducing the surgeon's professional fees.

SUMMARY

WALANT is well established in Brazil and is spreading rapidly. The authors have found many advantages to its use and continue to discover more. By applying fairness in surgeon reimbursement, Brazilian health plan insurers can help spread this technique, which decreases patient cost and improves patient safety and results of surgery.

REFERENCES

1. Bunnell S. Surgery of the hand. Philadelphia: Lippincott; 1944.
2. Bunnell S, Boyes JH. Principios de reconstruccíon. In: Bunnell S, Boyes JH, editors. Cirurgia de la mano. Buenos Aires (Argentina): Inter-Medica; 1967. p. 119–47.
3. Lalonde DH, Bell M, Benoit P, et al. A multicenter prospective study of 3,110 consecutive case of elective epinephrine use in the fingers and hand:

the Dalhousie project clinical phase. J Hand Surg Am 2005;30:1061–7.

4. Chowdhry S, Seidenstriker L, Cooney DS, et al. Do not use epinephrine in digital blocks: myth or truth? Part II. A retrospective review of 1111 cases. Plast Reconstr Surg 2010;126:2031–4.

5. Sardenberg T, Ribak S, Colenci R, et al. 488 cirurgias da mão com anestesia local com epinefrina, sem torniquete, sem sedação e sem anestesista. Rev Bras Ortop 2018;53:281–6.

6. Novais Junior RAFN, Costa BRJ, Carmo JMMC. Uso de adrenalina com lidocaina em cirurgia da mão. Rev Bras Ortop 2013;49:452–60.

7. Barros MFFH, Luz Junior AR, Roncaglio B, et al. Avaliação do tratamento cirúrgico da síndrome do túnel do carpo com anestesia local. Rev Bras Ortop 2016;51:36–9.

8. Lalonde DH. Safe epinephrine in the finger means no torniquete. In: Lalonde DH, editor. Wide awake hand surgery. Boca Raton (FL): CRC Press; 2016. p. 23–8.

9. Pires Neto PJ. Anatomia patológica da sinóvia de pacientes submetidos à liberação do túnel do carpo. Acta Ortop Bras 2010;18:200–3.

10. Pires Neto PJ, Moreira LA, Las Casas PP. É seguro o uso de anestésico local com adrenalina na cirurgia da mão? Técnica WALANT. Rev Bras Ortop 2017; 52:383–9.

11. Lalonde DH. Conceptual origins, current practice, and views of wide awake hand surgery. J Hand Surg Eur Vol 2017;42:886–95.

Lessons Learned in the Authors' First Years of Wide-Awake Hand Surgery at the W Hospital in Korea

Sang Hyun Woo, MD, PhD*, Myung Jae Yoo, MD,
Hee Chan Ahn, MD

KEYWORDS

• Wide-awake surgery • W hospital • Korea • WALANT

KEY POINTS

- Since 2017, the application of wide-awake local anesthesia no tourniquet (WALANT) surgery in Korea has greatly increased because of reduced costs and improved operation outcomes.
- The authors have mainly used WALANT in tendon surgery and have been impressed that intraoperative active movement examination by awake patients has helped them get better results.
- The use of local anesthesia instead of ultrasound-guided brachial plexus block reduces the money a hospital can receive under the current medical insurance system.
- Although WALANT is better for patients, a modification to the medical payment system is needed to motivate anesthesiologists to use the technique.

INTRODUCTION

Putting patients under sedation incurs a greater cost to both patients and practice and increases the time required for preoperative testing and consultation as well as postoperative recovery and care. It also increases the inconvenience for patients because of the need to fast before the operation and the lengthy time the whole procedure and recovery takes. The surgeon also experiences the inconvenience of being unable to communicate with patients midoperation to get feedback on patients' active range of motion in real time. Wide-awake local anesthesia no tourniquet (WALANT) surgery addresses these drawbacks.

THE BEGINNING OF WIDE-AWAKE HAND SURGERY IN KOREA

Even though most Korean hand surgeons are aware of WALANT surgery and are very interested in it, the clinical applications of this technique have been very limited to date. With no published articles in the official journal of the Korean Society for Surgery of the Hand and no presentations at the annual meeting until 2016, the motivation for surgeons to learn and adopt the technique was minimal. At the annual meeting in 2016, there were only 2 presentations on WALANT among a total of 105 presentations. In 2017, this number only increased to a total of 4 among 100 free articles.

Disclosure Statement: The authors have nothing to disclose.
W Institute for Hand & Reconstructive Microsurgery, W General Hospital, 1632 Dalgubeol-daero, Dalseo-Gu, Daegu 42642, Korea
* Corresponding author.
E-mail address: handwoo@hotmail.com

Hand Clin 35 (2019) 59–66
https://doi.org/10.1016/j.hcl.2018.08.006

In 2016, Dr Lalonde was invited to speak in 4 Korean cities as well as at the annual national hand surgery meeting by this article's first author (S.H. Woo). Dr Lalonde gave a keynote lecture on "How Wide Awake Hand Surgery is Improving Results and Decreasing Complications" to Korean hand surgeons. These opportunities were organized by Dr Woo, who was first introduced to WALANT at the Indonesian instruction course of hand surgery in Jakarta in May 2015. All 7 invited professors from overseas, including Dr Lalonde, spoke about topics on hand surgery to Indonesian doctors. At that time, Dr Lalonde convincingly demonstrated how the WALANT technique can be painless and how intraoperative patient education can be helpful to decrease complications. He dispelled the danger myths related to epinephrine's vasoconstrictive effects. All attendees were very impressed by the new horizons offered by the WALANT technique. Dr Woo also subsequently arranged for his colleague (H.C. Ahn) to visit Dr Lalonde's clinic for observation of WALANT in Canada.

WIDE-AWAKE HAND SURGERY AT W HOSPITAL

The Korean Ministry of Health and Welfare has designated 4 hospitals as specialty centers for replantation surgery in Korea, including W hospital, which is one of the biggest private centers for hand and reconstructive microsurgery in Korea. It has 260 beds, and there are 10 hand surgery specialists working together in 8 operation rooms in a single building.

Originally, almost all cases of hand and upper extremity surgery were performed with ultrasound-guided axillary block anesthesia except for some cases of congenital surgery for babies. After recognizing the effectiveness of wide-awake hand surgery, the authors began to use this technique more often. According to the annual reports of W hospital in 2016 and 2017, the total number of hand surgeries was around 12,500 and 13,900 cases, respectively. Among them, the number of wide-awake hand surgeries was 136 and 293. Most are related to tendon problems (**Table 1**). The number of wide-awake hand surgeries in 2017 has increased dramatically.

According to recent reports, the WALANT technique can be applied to many aspects of hand surgery, including primary and secondary tendon reconstruction, wrist arthroscopy, peripheral nerve compression, operative fixation of metacarpal and phalangeal fractures, trapeziectomy, and release of Dupuytren contracture.[1–7] Flap or replantation may not be a contraindication for this technique,

as demonstrated in Shu Guo Xing and Jin Bo Tang's article, "Extending Applications of Local Anesthesia Without Tourniquet to Flap Harvest and Transfer in the Hand," in this issue. This technique is even used for forefoot and ankle surgery.[8,9] Indications of the WALANT technique are currently widening from tendons to nerve, bone, joints, as well as from distal parts of the hand to proximal parts of upper extremities.

Despite the many advantages, the indication for WALANT at W hospital have been limited to tendon surgery in the authors' beginning. Primary repair of flexor and extensor tendon lacerations is the first and the most common indication. Secondary tenolysis of tendons, tendon graft, or tendon transfers in delayed reconstruction of flexor or extensor tendon are recognized as also good indications in the authors' practice. The authors are also now doing some cases of complex tendon transfers for median, radial, and ulnar palsy under wide-awake anesthesia. Recently, the authors have added surgery for congenital camptodactyly as well as trigger fingers. The authors have also begun to perform cases of arthrodesis and hand fracture surgery under wide-awake anesthesia.

MODIFICATIONS OF WIDE-AWAKE HAND SURGERY AT W HOSPITAL

WALANT hand surgery has many advantages,[10] including lower costs to patients, more efficient workflow in the operating room, simpler surgical draping, reduced operating time through omission of the tourniquet, and elimination of the need for conventional postoperative recovery. During the operation, patients can see and demonstrate active movement to the surgeons. Surgeons can advise patients about their postoperative care. By reducing garbage production with simpler draping of operative field, WALANT is contributing to the greening of surgery for a better environment.

Although there are many advantages of the WALANT technique, there are some limitations for doctors. The main limiting factor in Korea is that the national insurance system does not yet allow or accept medical expenses for local anesthetic injection for WALANT. This circumstance is why the authors have modified the WALANT technique.

Who Administers Injections?

Previous anesthesia for hand surgery at W hospital was almost all performed under ultrasound-guided brachial plexus block by 3 anesthesiologists who are all full-time employees of the hospital. Because the success rate of this method of anesthesia is

Table 1
Wide-awake tendon surgery in the hand in 2016 and 2017 at W hospital

Procedures	Tendons	2016		2017	
		Wide Awake	Non–Wide Awake	Wide Awake	Non–Wide Awake
Primary repair	Flexor	36 (13.4%)	232 (86.6%)	75 (23.5%)	244 (76.5%)
	Extensor	37 (5.3%)	662 (94.7%)	77 (9.9%)	704 (90.1%)
Tenolysis	Flexor	28 (37.8%)	46 (62.2%)	67 (55.8%)	53 (44.2%)
	Extensor	16 (26.7%)	44 (73.3%)	28 (47.5%)	31 (52.5%)
Transfer	Flexor	4 (22.2%)	14 (77.8%)	21 (70.0%)	9 (30.0%)
	Extensor	15 (44.1%)	19 (55.9%)	25 (65.8%)	13 (34.2%)

more than 98%,[11] general endotracheal anesthesia for the surgery is mostly limited to congenital cases in infants and patients of preschool age. All anesthesiologists always try to perform a nerve block first.

In all cases of wide-awake hand surgery, the 3 anesthesiologists inject the local anesthesia instead of the surgeons. When surgeons get informed consent for the operation, they draw the area for the expected area of incision and dissection on the finger or hand. The anesthesiologist then injects lidocaine and epinephrine in the drawn area of dissection in the recovery room where patients are lying on a stretcher. They usually finish injections 20 to 30 minutes before the operation. This preparation of anesthesia increases the efficiency and utility rate of the operation room. Sometimes the anesthesiologist complains of pain and weakness of their hands after large-volume injections for large operative fields with small-gauge needles. Without any burden of anesthesia, the surgeons can concentrate on the operation itself.

Wide-Awake Local Anesthesia with a Brief Tourniquet Period

The original WALANT technique has many advantages for patients as well as surgeons as described in previous articles. At W hospital, one modification is wide-awake local anesthesia with a brief tourniquet period. The authors find that the tumescent tissues and bleeding in the operative field interfere with the initial meticulous dissection of important or vital structures. The authors, therefore, inflate an arm tourniquet for 3 to 20 minutes to perform the initial dissection. The duration of tourniquet application varies depending on the patients' tolerance for pain. The authors have observed that the patients can endure about 14 minutes on average. This time is enough for the surgeon to incise the skin and dissect the important structures. Whenever patients complain of pain,

the tourniquet is deflated. Whenever the authors need a clear or bloodless field during any operative steps, the tourniquet is inflated again for 5 to 10 minutes. The authors do not insist on no tourniquet, but they do not want to hurt patients.

Sedation

WALANT is safer for patients than sedation, especially for individuals with medical comorbidities. The safest sedation is no sedation.[12] It also helps to eliminate the rare occasion when surgeons operate on the wrong hand or finger because awake patients are more likely to point out the error than those who are sedated. However, some patients want to be asleep during the operation and they do not want to hear anything, including beeps from the echocardiogram or monitor of oxygen saturation inside the operation room. In these cases, the authors give small doses of a sedative, such as a benzodiazepine. Then, the authors can wake patients to assess active movement of the finger and wrist as part of tendon surgery or fracture reduction. The authors would not insist on no sedation for the patients who want to be asleep.

Open Communication

In cases of general endotracheal anesthesia, it is not possible to educate patients about the surgery and postoperative care during the surgery. Even after surgery, patients have not sufficiently recovered from the anesthesia to understand the surgeon's recommendations or postoperative instructions in the recovery room. They cannot remember what the surgeon told them because of amnestic medications.

The elimination of general anesthesia with WALANT is, thus, an enormous benefit for patients' education and understanding.[9] Surgeons can inform patients about postoperative care during the operation to avoid postoperative complications. The authors always recommend to their patients that they should look to see their movement after the repair of structures during the surgery. Seeing helps them remember how their hand or fingers can move after the authors have mended the defects. They can also completely understand what they need to do for a successful recovery. From the start, patients become an active participant in the rehabilitation team with the surgeon and even the therapist.

The authors' early clinical experiences have demonstrated that intraoperative active motion of the digits or hand is not always maintained at long-term follow-up. Some patients are disappointed by a long-term result that is not as good as what they saw during surgery. Reasons for this include the normal wound-healing processes, postoperative pain, and a possibly unexpected course during and after rehabilitation. Therefore, when the surgeon shows the range of motion of the hand or digits to patients intraoperatively, the authors should explain the possibility of a less satisfactory long-term result. The authors now always say the following: The range of motion of your reconstructed tendon is the best it can be right now. If you want to maintain this active motion, you must follow postoperative rehabilitation diligently. The wound-healing process may lessen or worsen the movement you have right now.

LESSONS LEARNED IN WIDE-AWAKE FLEXOR TENDON REPAIR

In the past, in primary repair of flexor tendons, the authors have concentrated more on how many strands and what repair technique is sufficiently strong to prevent rupture or reduce adhesion of repaired tendon by early active exercise. Repaired, and thereby thickened, flexor tendons are not able to move freely in a repaired tendon sheath, because of the increased diameter of the repaired tendon or narrowing of the sheath by the process of closing it.

Since the authors started wide-awake tendon surgery, the most important thing they have learned is that it increases the surgeons' confidence in the operation. The authors can directly observe and repair gapping of the sutured tendons gliding under the pulley when they test active range of motion of the digits before skin closure (**Fig. 1**). Complete closure of the sheath used to result in complete or partial immobility of the repair and was more likely to cause snagging with movement. The authors now vent the pulleys as required depending on both the active range of motion and the bowstringing effect. The repeated full active motion of repaired tendon verifies that the repair is strong and that the pulley release is sufficient. With wide-awake anesthesia, the name *no man's land* in flexor tendon injury at zone 2 has surely become *young man's land*.

Wide-awake flexor tendon repair reduces tendon rupture rates.[13–15] The authors have not yet proven this with evidence-based data from their own clinical experience, but they do think this is the case. In the future, they plan to verify the relationship between the amount of venting of each pulley and improvement of the range of motion of each joint and the comparison of the incidence rate of rupture and adhesion with and without wide-awake anesthesia based on their clinical experiences.

LESSONS LEARNED IN WIDE-AWAKE TENDON TRANSFER

In flexor tendon transfer for secondary reconstruction, wide-awake surgery is the best option (**Fig. 2**) because adjusting the tension of the transfer has always proven difficult under brachial plexus block or general anesthesia.[16] With patients being awake, the digits or the hand can move actively to determine the correct tension of the transfer. Surgeons can check appropriate tension of the reconstructed tendon as well as the gliding status during the operation. The concerns about making the transfer too tight or too loose are eliminated. It is also possible for the surgeon to check gap formation even in repeated strong grip during the procedure to eliminate the risk of postoperative rupture.

In cases of late low radial nerve palsy, defined as an injury to the posterior interosseous nerve, tendon transfer is the best option for reconstruction (see **Fig. 2**). The amount of passive tension at which the tendon transfer procedure is set is the most critical aspect of the operation. To achieve maximum force generation, the muscle must be set at an optimum degree of tension. With wide-awake anesthesia, the surgeon can feel the most appropriate tension intraoperatively depending on the position of the adjacent joints. The tendon transfer juncture tends to relax and lengthen postoperatively, and a transfer that is set with inadequate tension will not improve with time.

With these cases, the authors were initially concerned about the large volume and the effect of local injection of the lidocaine and epinephrine for large and deep areas of injection. They now inject diluted 0.5% lidocaine with 1:200,000 epinephrine to decrease the total amount of injected epinephrine, which has both strong anesthetic and vasoconstrictive effects.

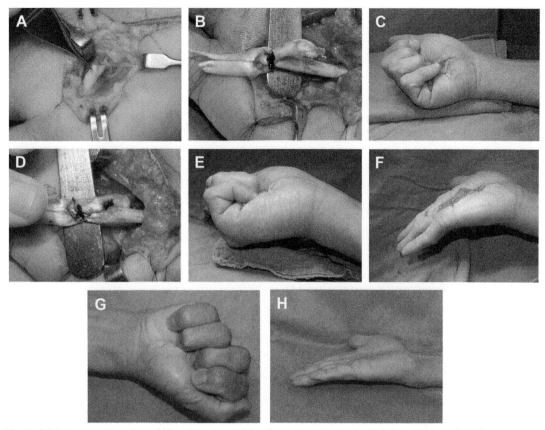

Fig. 1. (*A*) Intraoperative view of closed rupture of the flexor tendons to the right small finger. Attritional rupture of the fifth flexor digitorum profundus tendon at zone III. (*B, C*) Temporary suturing between the fourth flexor digitorum sublimis tendon does not provide full flexion of the distal interphalangeal (DIP) joint. (*D, E*) Readjustment of tension with shortening about 1.5 cm makes the small finger flex the DIP joint more. (*F*) Intraoperative view shows full extension of the ring and small fingers after tendon repair with the Pulvertaft technique. (*G, H*) Postoperative view, 13 months later.

LESSONS LEARNED IN WIDE-AWAKE TENOLYSIS

Tenolysis of the digits can be done with similar anesthesia under short or no tourniquet techniques (**Fig. 3**). Patients can actively move the digits or hand to ensure that the tenolysis has been adequate and that the tendon is strong enough to move the tendon. Even in combined reconstruction of the pulley with tenolysis, the surgeon avoids complications by checking the gliding of the tendon that has undergone tenolysis under the new pulley. If the tenolysis is insufficient, the surgeon can conduct further release of the tendon, joint, or scar contracture. If active movement is still not full despite further release, the surgeon can check tendon adhesion more proximally or distally.

After testing strong flexion, the surgeon can decide to shorten or strengthen the frayed tendon immediately if it seems inadequate. The authors have observed that in complicated tenolysis and contracture release of combined joint and tendon problems together, long-term postoperative movement can be inferior to the intraoperative range of motion. Previous complex injury, such as digital amputation or severe crushing injuries, frequently have relatively bad results after secondary surgery, even under wide-awake anesthesia.

LESSONS LEARNED IN EXTENSOR TENDON REPAIR

Surgeons experience less difficulty in wide-awake extensor surgery than in wide-awake flexor tendon surgery. In extensor tendon injuries, each component of the extensor tendon over the fingers tolerates little loss of tendon substance. In repairing the extensor tendon, gliding and strength of repaired tendon is not as important as it is for flexor tendons.

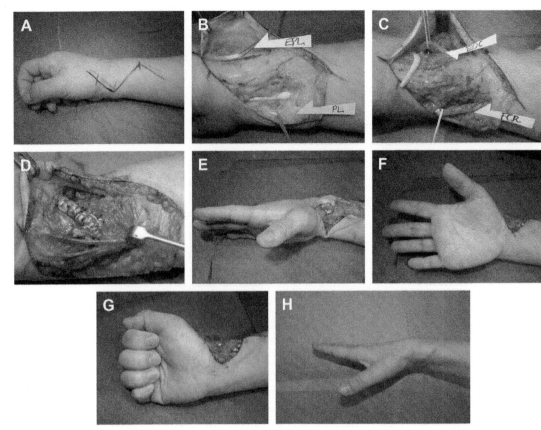

Fig. 2. (*A*) A 52-year-old woman had posterior interosseous neuropathy of the right forearm for 6 years. (*B*) Around one incision over the radio-dorsal wrist, 0.5% 50 mL lidocaine with 1:200,000 epinephrine was used to decrease the total amount of injected epinephrine. (*B*) Skin incision and dissection of both the palmaris longus (PL) tendon and extensor pollicis longus (EPL) tendon is performed under tourniquet. (*C*) Two tendons of flexor carpi radialis (FCR) and extensor digitorum communis (EDC) are dissected without a tourniquet. (*D*) Interweaving sutures are made PL to EPL and FCR to EDC with adjusting tension. (*E–G*) Intraoperative assessment of the motion after tendon transfer. (*H*) Finger and thumb extension 15 months later.

LESSONS LEARNED FROM INTRAOPERATIVE PATIENT EDUCATION

The authors have observed that patients are definitely more cooperative toward the rehabilitation program because they have already seen their active motion during the surgery. During the operation, they have been educated to become actively involved in the rehabilitation program. This involvement is more likely to guarantee favorable postoperative satisfaction.

LESSONS LEARNED FROM REPLANTATION OR REVASCULARIZATION OF DIGITS

Because the possibility of using this approach in flap surgery and replantation was reported,[17,18] in some cases of incomplete or complete replantation of the digits, the authors attempted wide-awake anesthesia. Even after radical debridement

of devitalized tissues, it was not easy to get strong pulsation of the proximal artery; the authors, therefore, hesitate to use this technique at this time. The operator may hesitate to further debride the amputated artery or not. Vasospasm of the vessel results from the amputation injury itself as well as possibly because of the vasoconstriction of the epinephrine.

MEDICAL EXPENSE AND INSURANCE PROBLEMS RELATED TO ANESTHESIA

The health insurance system in Korea is controlled by the government. All Korean people are required to sign up for this national insurance. The Ministry of Health and Welfare of Korea has an affiliated organization called the Health Insurance Review and Assessment (HIRA) service, which regulates and judges the charge of medical treatments by doctors. Medical fees related to hand surgery are still

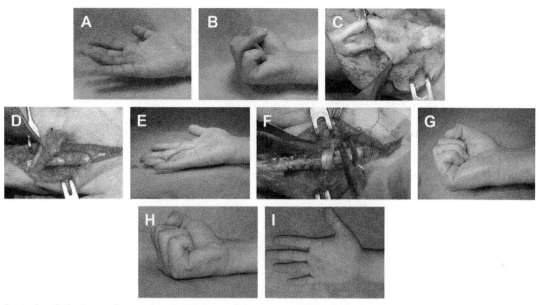

Fig. 3. (*A*, *B*) Flexion and extension contracture of the proximal interphalangeal (PIP) joint of the ring finger after flexor tendon repair. (*C*) After opening the tendon sheath, the authors found severe adhesions between the flexor digitorum sublimis (FDS) and flexor digitorum profundus (FDP) tendons as well as between flexor tendons and pulleys. (*D*) Tenolysis with FDS tendon tenotomy, capsulotomy, and volar plate release at the PIP joint resulted in active extension of the PIP joint. (*E*) Test of full digital extension during surgery. (*F*) FDP tendon was strengthened with a modified Becker method, and the A2 pulley was reconstructed with resected FDS remnant over the repaired FDP tendon. (*G*) Immediate postoperative view. (*H*, *I*) Postoperative view, full flexion and extension, 10 months later.

not paid by the prospective payment system, which is based on diagnosis-related groupings. The medical expense of the operation fee is only for the surgeon's activity. This point means that the anesthesiologist must contribute something inside the operation room for the all surgeries and surgeons. If not, it is not easy for anesthesiologists to get their salary from the hospital.

Even though all hand specialists of W hospital understand the many advantages of wide-awake hand surgery, the number of cases in 2017 was only 293, which is only 2.1% of all hand surgeries. There are economic reasons why the number of cases has not increased more. One is the anesthesia fee related to local injection by the surgeon. The operation fee under local anesthesia includes both the operative procedure as well as the local anesthesia injection. For example, if the carpal tunnel release is performed under local anesthesia, the operation fee is $253 (268,923 Korean Won, 1 USD = 1064 KRW) and $0.5 for the lidocaine. In this case, the hospital cannot claim the fee for the disposable operation drape set. If the surgeons do this operation under brachial plexus block, they can claim more fees for monitoring of oxygen saturation and anesthesia, which adds up to about $96

(101,736 KRW). If the anesthesiologist conducts an ultrasound-guided brachial plexus block, a further $66 (70,000 KRW) can be added. The total medical fee of the carpal tunnel release is 1.7 times higher under ultrasound-guided brachial plexus block than it is under local anesthesia. Fair reimbursement needs to evolve.

SOLUTIONS FOR INCREASING POPULARITY OF WIDE-AWAKE ANESTHESIA IN KOREA

Most anesthesiologists in Korea are not so interested in regional blocks or wide-awake anesthesia for hand surgery, especially for the hand. For patients, wide-awake anesthesia is the best way to perform operations because of convenience, risk, and reduced medical expenses. For these reasons, surgeons should be using the technique more often.

If the HIRA of the Korean government starts to adopt a prospective payment system based on diagnosis-related grouping as a medical expenses payment system, hand surgeons nationwide will adopt wide-awake surgery techniques without any hesitation. Doctors can reduce current expenditures on anesthesiologists, operation packs, and unnecessary laboratory studies. However, this will only be possible with the precondition that the operation fee would actually increase. This change in our national health insurance system would induce a change in doctors' routine behavior, which would be economically better for patients, surgeons, and the government.

Under the current tight health insurance system, the authors cannot give up the anesthesia fee for hand surgery. Wide-awake anesthesia could decrease the total medical expenses for the surgery as well as increase the safety of patients. In addition, the authors could contribute to the conservation of nature by reducing the resources consumed and the waste produced from surgery. All revenue savings from wide-awake anesthesia should return to the doctors. Public officers and all parties concerned with the national health insurance should pay attention to the invaluable advantages of wide-awake anesthesia. At the academic society level, both the Korean Society for Surgery of the Hand and the Korean Society of Anesthesiologists should create a new item of medical expense for wide-awake anesthesia for government adoption.

ACKNOWLEDGMENTS

The authors would like to thank Andrew J. Miller for proofreading and editing the text.

REFERENCES

1. Lalonde DH. Wide-awake extensor indicis proprius to extensor pollicis longus tendon transfer. J Hand Surg Am 2014;39:2297–9.
2. Tang JB. Wide-awake primary flexor tendon repair, tenolysis, and tendon transfer. Clin Orthop Surg 2015;7:275–81.
3. Hagert E, Lalonde DH. Wide-awake wrist arthroscopy and open TFCC repair. J Wrist Surg 2012;1:55–60.
4. Lalonde DH. Reconstruction of the hand with wide awake surgery. Clin Plast Surg 2011;38:761–9.
5. Lalonde DH. "Hole-in-one" local anesthesia for wide-awake carpal tunnel surgery. Plast Reconstr Surg 2010;126:1642–4.
6. Farhangkhoee H, Lalonde J, Lalonde DH. Wide-awake trapeziectomy: video detailing local anesthetic injection and surgery. Hand (N Y) 2011;6:466–7.
7. Nelson R, Higgins A, Conrad J, et al. The Wide-awake approach to Dupuytren's disease: fasciectomy under local anesthetic with epinephrine. Hand (N Y) 2010;5:117–24.
8. MacNeill AL, Mayich DJ. Wide-awake foot and ankle surgery: a retrospective analysis. Foot Ankle Surg 2017;23:307–10.
9. Wright J, MacNeill AL, Mayich DJ. A prospective comparison of wide-awake local anesthesia and general anesthesia for forefoot surgery. Foot Ankle Surg 2017;6 [pii:S1268-7731:31326-31327].
10. Tang JB, Gong KT, Zhu L, et al. Performing hand Surgery under local anesthesia without a tourniquet in China. Hand Clin 2017;33:415–24.
11. Seo BB, Kim YW, Woo SH. Comparison of axillary and supraclavicular approach in ultrasound-guided brachial plexus block. J Korean Soc Surg Hand 2014;19:130–5.
12. Lalonde DH. What is wide awake hand surgery? In: Wide awake hand surgery. New York: CRC Press; 2016. p. 17–22.
13. Higgins A, Lalonde DH, Bell M, et al. Avoiding flexor tendon repair rupture with intraoperative total active movement examination. Plast Reconstr Surg 2010;126:941–5.
14. Lalonde DH. Conceptual origins, current practice, and views of wide awake hand surgery. J Hand Surg Eur Vol 2017;42:886–95.
15. Gibson PD, Sobol GL, Ahmed IH. Zone II flexor tendon repairs in the United States: trends in current management. J Hand Surg Am 2017;42:99e–108e.
16. Woo SH, Lee YK, Kim JM, et al. Hand and wrist injuries in golfers and their treatment. Hand Clin 2017;33:81–96.
17. Xing SG, Mao T. The use of local anaesthesia with epinephrine in the harvest and transfer of an extended Segmuller flap in the fingers. J Hand Surg Eur 2018;43:783–4.
18. Wong J, Lin CH, Chang NJ, et al. Digital revascularization and replantation using the wide-awake hand surgery technique. J Hand Surg Eur Vol 2017;42:621–5.

Wide Awake Tendon Transfers in Leprosy Patients in India

Akbar Khan Mohammed, MS[a,*],
Donald H. Lalonde, MSc, DSc, MD, FRCSC[b]

KEYWORDS

- WALANT • Hand reconstructive surgery in leprosy • Tendon transfer in leprosy • Affordable surgery
- Safe epinephrine in finger

KEY POINTS

- Wide awake local anesthesia no tourniquet (WALANT) with tumescent local anesthesia in reconstructive surgeries in hand in leprosy is a good alternative to tourniquet anesthesia.
- WALANT provides effective anesthesia with good visibility for leprosy tendon transfers.
- WALANT permits economically disadvantaged leprosy patients to afford the surgery.
- All of the leprosy patients who have undergone WALANT tendon transfers in this series would like the same technique for their next tendon transfers.

Leprosy causes peripheral nerve paralysis that leads to tendon imbalances in the wrist, hand, and fingers. Paul Brand began some of the history of human tendon transfer surgery on leprosy patients in India. It is still a problem that is more prevalent in patients who can frequently not easily afford reconstructive surgery. The recent advances in wide awake surgery have eliminated the need for expensive anesthesiology drugs, equipment, and personnel. This article examines early experience using wide awake local anesthesia no tourniquet (WALANT) technique in leprosy patients in Nellore, India.

Dr Akbar Khan observed Dr Don Lalonde operate and speak on WALANT hand surgery July 3-5, 2015 at Ganga Hospital, in Coimbatore India. Dr Khan began using the technique shortly thereafter at the Damien Foundation Hospital in Nellore, India.

Before this, he performed leprosy hand surgery under axillary block with a tourniquet. Dr Khan finds the technique has many advantages, including increased safety and affordability in this population. This article summarizes his first 18 months of experience and describes 5 of his operations.

TUMESCENT LOCAL MIXTURES FOR LEPROSY SURGERY

Tumescence is the injection of dilute lidocaine and epinephrine into the subcutaneous tissue wherever one is going to cut or dissect.[1] The classic tumescent anesthesia described by Klein,[2] with a standard formula of 0.05% lidocaine and 1:1,000,000 epinephrine plus sodium bicarbonate (8.4%) in 1 L of saline (0.9%), works well for liposuction procedures. The lidocaine is for anesthesia, and the

---

Disclosure Statement: Dr A.K. Mohammed has no disclosures. Dr D.H. Lalonde is the editor of the book *Wide Awake Hand Surgery* (Thieme publishers) 2016. He makes no profit on the sales of the book. All royalties go to the American Association for Hand Surgery Lean and Green effort, which is dedicated to decreasing unnecessary cost and garbage production in hand surgery. He otherwise has no disclosures.

[a] Orthopedics, Damien Foundation Hospital, Bhakthavatsala Nagar, Nellore, Andhra Pradesh 524004, India;
[b] Division of Plastic Surgery, Dalhousie University, Dalhousie Medicine New Brunswick, Suite C204, 600 Main Street, Saint John, New Brunswick E2K 1J5, Canada
* Corresponding author.
E-mail address: akbarmast@gmail.com

Hand Clin 35 (2019) 67–84
https://doi.org/10.1016/j.hcl.2018.09.001

epinephrine provides hemostasis instead of the tourniquet. The basic principle common to all techniques is the delivery of a large amount of fluid with a local anesthetic and a vasoconstrictor. This technique results in swelling or tumescence of the operative field.[3] There have been many modifications. Prasetyono uses 1:1,000,000 epinephrine for his tumescent solution for hand surgery.[4]

The advantages of tumescent technique have been well published within the literature. They include shorter surgical times, less postoperative edema, reduced risk of hematomas, improved postoperative pain control, and avoidance of general anesthetic. In addition, when infiltrated at the appropriate depth, the tumescent solution acts as a natural hydro-dissector, creating avascular anatomic tissue planes for easier and more rapid dissection.[5]

Tumescent local anesthesia is like a tourniquet-free extravascular Bier block in which lidocaine with epinephrine is injected subcutaneously only where it is needed.[6] The authors' basic solution before dilution in Nellore contains 1% lidocaine, 1:100,000 epinephrine, and 8.4% bicarbonate. They make this with the locally available Lidocaine 2%, adrenaline 1:1000, and sodium bicarbonate 7.5%. They keep the total dose of lidocaine less than 7 mg/kg. The average 60-kg person can, therefore, safely receive 45 mL of 1% lidocaine with epinephrine.

PREPARATION OF TUMESCENT LOCAL ANESTHESIA SOLUTION IN NELLORE, INDIA

If 45 mL is required, the authors use 20 mL of 2% lidocaine dilute with 20 mL normal saline (that makes a total of 40 mL), add 0.4 mL of adrenaline (to make 1:1000–1:1,00,000), and add 4.8 mL of 7.5% $NaHCO_3$ (as 1 mL of 8.3% $NAHCO_3$ for each 10 mL of 1% lidocaine) (**Table 1**).

If 50 to 100 mL will be required (hand and forearm cases), the authors dilute the local with saline (50:50) to a mixture of 0.5% lidocaine with 1:200,000 epinephrine. In large forearm cases that need a volume of 100 to 200 mL to anesthetize a large area, the authors use 0.25% lidocaine with 1:400,000 epinephrine.

The authors start by injecting a large volume in the most proximal location that any dissection is likely to take place to block the nerves distally. The end point of effective tumescent anesthetic infiltration is pale and firm skin with visible and palpable local anesthesia beneath it.

LEPROSY SURGERY EXPERIENCE

This prospective study was conducted at the Damien Foundation Hospital from July 2015 to December 2017 in which the authors performed 56 reconstructive surgeries for deformities in the hand in leprosy. The authors injected freshly prepared mixtures of local anesthetic in their patients on stretchers in their outpatient department 30 minutes before moving the patient to the theater to perform the surgery. The authors counseled the patient about the administration of anesthesia, the operative procedure, and the postoperative care and physiotherapy.

After their surgery, the authors asked patients to give their preferences of anesthesia technique for their future operations. Most of these patients have multiple deformities because of several nerve palsies due to leprosy. Most of them had already been through procedures with brachial plexus block in the past and would need more surgery in the future. The authors evaluated pain while injecting the local anesthesia and during the operative procedure with visual analogue scales. They also measured the volume infiltration of infiltrated local anesthesia solution and estimated the amount of bleeding in the surgical field. The authors recorded the operative time for each procedure as well as the complications. They noted the advantages and disadvantages during the procedures as well as the patient feedback and their preferences (**Fig. 1**). The data are described in **Table 2**.

The following text details 5 procedures for which wide awake surgery was performed in this unit.

DIRECT LASSO PROCEDURE

Transfer of flexor digitorum superficialis (FDS) of middle finger transfer into 4 finger flexor A1 and A2 pulleys for claw hand deformities is shown in **Fig. 2**.

Local Anesthetic Technique

The images of the local anesthetic injection sites in **Fig. 3** are those of a normal hand, not a claw hand. In the waiting area outside the operating room, the authors cleaned the hand. Five milliliters of tumescent local anesthesia was infiltrated in the proximal flexion crease in the proximal interphalangeal (PIP) joint of middle finger without letting the needle advance beyond 3 to 4 mm of the white tumesced subcutaneous tissue. Eight to 10 mL of solution was then injected longitudinally from proximal to distal starting just distal to the flexor retinaculum along midline of the palm. Each of the 4 fingers were then injected with 5 mL at the metacarpophalangeal (MP) joints. More than 30 minutes later, surgery began in the operating room after moving the patient to that location. This delay gave the epinephrine ample time to work properly.

Comment by Dr Lalonde

It may be less painful to inject the proximal palm first and then inject 10 mL in one injection between the index and middle MP joints, followed by 10 mL in one injection between the ring and small MP joints. The last injection would be in the long finger, where it may be less painful to inject 2 mL in the subcutaneous fat of the midline of the proximal phalanx followed by 2 mL in the subcutaneous fat of the midline of the middle phalanx. The 2 distal palm and the 2 finger injections would be just under the skin without moving the needle.

SURGICAL PROCEDURE

The following text describes what is seen in the images in **Fig. 4**.

A 1- to 1.5-cm incision was made in the volar crease of the PIP joint of the middle finger. The flexor digitorum profundus (FDP) was identified (see **Fig. 4**A) and retracted radially and then ulnarly to detach the 2 slips of FDS from their insertion. The 2 slips were separated at the chiasm (see **Fig. 4**B).

A 2-cm longitudinal incision was made just distal to the flexor retinaculum (transverse carpal ligament) along the midline. The authors split the palmar aponeurosis and opened the flexor synovial sheath. The authors identified FDS of long finger and delivered it outside the incision (see **Fig. 4**C). They split the 2 slips up to below the incision and then divided both slips into 2 tails so they had 4 tails of FDS tendon powered by the FDS muscle. They could now test the active excursion of FDS in the awake, comfortable tourniquet-free patient if the authors were unsure of its power and excursion.

The authors made a curved incision connecting the radial end of middle palmar crease and the ulnar end of distal palmar crease. They developed flaps containing skin and subcutaneous fat distally up to the base of the fingers and proximally up to 1 cm to expose the A1 and A2 pulleys of each finger (see **Fig. 4**D). The authors passed an Anderson tunneller or a curved artery forceps from the distal palmar incision through the radial interosseous space into the proximal longitudinal incision to pull each of the 4 tails through to each MP joint in the palmar incision (see **Fig. 4**E). The authors closed the finger and proximal palm incisions (see **Fig. 4**F). In **Fig. 4**F, there is a second proximal incision at the base of the thumb through which a Z deformity of the thumb was also corrected in this case.

The authors took the tip of a tendon tail with end of a mosquito forceps or a guide eye tunneler and passed it through the flexor tunnel to bring it out through middle of the A2 pulley (see **Fig. 4**G). They then passed the other 3 tails through their respective flexor tunnels. They folded the tails back over the proximal half of A2 and A1 pulley in the right tension and fixed them to themselves proximal to the pulley with 2 or 3 sutures (see **Fig. 4**H). The authors began with the little finger where they applied maximum tension with the MP joint at 90°. They decreased the MP angle in each finger by 10° as they went to the index finger to maintain the cascade (see **Fig. 4**I). Then, the authors closed the incisions.

Comment from Dr Lalonde

At this point, I would get the patient to flex and extend all fingers to test the tension of the tendon transfer and make sure it is correct in all 4 fingers. I could adjust or reinforce my sutures if necessary, before closing the skin.

The authors applied a short arm cast for 3 weeks to keep the wrist neutral, MP joints flexed, and interphalangeal joints extended (**Fig. 5**).

Table 1
Mixtures of bicarbonate, epinephrine, and lidocaine

Total Solution Required (mL)	2% Lidocaine (mL)	Normal Saline (mL)	1:1000 Adrenaline, mL (1 mg/mL)	7.5% $NaHCO_3$ (mL)	Total Solution It Becomes (mL)
—	1	1	0.01	0.12	—
10	5	5	0.1	1.2	11.3
20	10	10	0.2	2.4	22.6
40	20	20	0.4	4.8	45.2

QUESTIONNAIRE FOR THE STUDY

Registration No.:_____

Name: _____

Age: _____ **Sex:** _____ **Weight:** _____ kg

Address: _____

Date of surgery: _____

Surgical procedure: _____

Amount of anesthetic solution (mL): _____

Operative time: _____

Pain during injection of local anesthesia: Visual Analogue Scale

Perioperative pain: Visual Analogue Scale

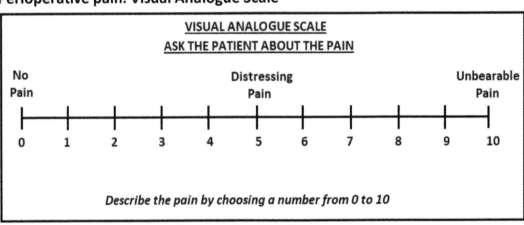

Perioperative bleeding: Excessive ( ) Moderate ( ) Minimal ( )

• Excessive: halts progression of the surgery unless a tourniquet is used

• Moderate: small amount oozing which could be stopped by mop compression

• Minimal: bleeding similar to that of surgery with a tourniquet

Complications: _____

WALANT technique preferred for next procedure: _____

Fig. 1. Data collected from each patient in the 18 months of data collection.

Indirect Lasso Procedure

Transfer of palmaris longus (PL) was extended with fascia lata into A1 and A2 flexor pulleys.

LOCAL ANESTHETIC TECHNIQUE

The images of the local anesthetic injection sites in **Fig. 6** are those of a normal hand, not a claw hand. In the waiting area outside the operating room, the authors cleaned the thigh for numbing the fascia lata donor site. They infiltrated enough local anesthesia solution from proximal to distal so that they could see it and feel it 2 cm beyond wherever they would incise or dissect. After cleaning the hand and forearm, the authors infiltrated 5 mL of local anesthesia at the middle of the proximal wrist crease at the palmaris longus insertion. They then infiltrated 5 mL of solution in the middle of the volar aspect of the forearm 5 cm above the proximal wrist crease. The authors then injected 8 to 10 mL of solution longitudinally from proximal to distal starting just distal to the flexor retinaculum along the midline of the palm. For the distal palm

Table 2
Data collected from the first 56 patients who underwent surgeries using the wide awake local anesthesia no tourniquet technique in the years 2015 to 2017 at the Damien Foundation Hospital, Nellore, India

Sample No.	Sex	Age	Type of Surgery	Amount of Solution, mL	Pain During Injection of LA (VAS Scale)	Operative Time	Perioperative Pain (VAS Scale)	Bleeding	Complications	WALANT Technique Preferred for Next Procedure
1	M	45	Right ulnar nerve decompression	20–25	4	1 h	2	Minimal	Nil	Yes
2	M	30	Right $\frac{1}{2}$ FPL to EPL	15	2	45 min	0	Minimal	Nil	Yes
3	F	19	Contracture release & thick skin graft	30	2	1 $\frac{1}{2}$ h	0	Minimal	Nil	Yes
4	F	42	Left $\frac{1}{2}$ FPL to EPL	15	2	45 min	0	Minimal	Nil	Yes
5	F	18	Left $\frac{1}{2}$ FPL to EPL	15	2	45 min	0	Minimal	Nil	Yes
6	M	45	Contracture release & thick skin graft	10	2	45 h	0	Minimal	Nil	Yes
7	M	60	Contracture release & thick skin graft	40	2	2 h	2	Minimal	Nil	Yes
8	M	14	Left ulnar nerve decompression	20–25	2	1 h	2	Moderate	Nil	Yes
9	M	19	Contracture release & thick skin graft	15	2	45 min	0	Minimal	Nil	Yes
10	M	20	Contracture release & thick skin graft	10	2	45 h	0	Minimal	Nil	Yes
11	M	30	Right ulnar nerve decompression	20–25	4	1 h	2	Minimal	Nil	Yes
12	F	43	Right S3 PI (2–5)	30	4	2 h	0	Minimal	Nil	Yes
13	F	24	Left S3 PI (2–5)	30	4	2 h	0	Minimal	Nil	Yes
14	F	41	Right S3 PI (2–5)	30	2	2 h	0	Minimal	Nil	Yes
15	M	30	Left S3 PI (2–5)	30	2	2 h	0	Minimal	Nil	Yes
16	M	62	Left S3 PI (2–5)	30	2	2 h	0	Minimal	Nil	Yes
17	M	35	Right S3 PI (2–5)	30	4	2 h	0	Minimal	Nil	Yes
18	M	20	Left S3 PI (2–5)	30	2	2 h	0	Minimal	Nil	Yes

(continued on next page)

Table 2
(continued)

Sample No.	Sex	Age	Type of Surgery	Amount of Solution, mL	Pain During Injection of LA (VAS Scale)	Operative Time	Perioperative Pain (VAS Scale)	Bleeding	Complications	WALANT Technique Preferred for Next Procedure
19	M	18	Left S3 PI (2–5) with 1/2 FPL to EPL	45	4	2½ h	2	Moderate	Nil	Yes
20	M	41	Left S3 PI (2–5)	30	2	2 h	0	Minimal	Nil	Yes
21	M	25	Right S3 PI (2–5)	30	2	2 h	0	Minimal	Nil	Yes
22	M	25	Left S3 PI (2–5)	30	2	2 h	0	Minimal	Nil	Yes
23	F	15	Left median nerve decompression	20–25	4	1 h	2	Minimal	Nil	Yes
24	M	35	Right S3 PI (2–5) with 1/2 FPL to EPL	45	2	2½ h	0	Moderate	Nil	Yes
25	M	35	Left S4 to thumb	30	2	1½ h	0	Minimal	Nil	Yes
26	M	17	Left ulnar nerve decompression	20–25	4	1 h	2	Moderate	Nil	Yes
27	M	14	Right radial nerve decompression	20–25	4	1 h	2	Moderate	Nil	Yes
28	M	35	Right S3 PI (2–5) with 1/2 FPL to EPL	45	4	2½ h	0	Minimal	Nil	Yes
29	M	40	Left S3 PI (2–5)	30	2	2 h	0	Minimal	Nil	Yes
30	M	25	Right S4 to Thumb	30	4	1½ h	0	Minimal	Nil	Yes
31	M	30	Left S3 PI (2–5) with 1/2 FPL to EPL	45	2	2½ h	0	Minimal	Nil	Yes
32	M	40	Left S3 PI (2–5)	30	2	2 h	0	Minimal	Nil	Yes
33	M	30	Right S3 PI (2–5)	30	2	2 h	0	Minimal	Nil	Yes
34	M	40	Left S3 PI (2–5)	30	2	2 h	0	Minimal	Nil	Yes
35	F	17	Left PL PI (2–5)	60	2	3 h	2	Moderate	Nil	Yes
36	F	42	Right S3 PI (2–5)	30	4	2 h	0	Minimal	Nil	Yes
37	M	21	Right PL PI (2–5)	60	4	3 h	2	Moderate	Nil	Yes
38	M	40	Left S4 to Thumb	30	4	1½ h	0	Minimal	Nil	Yes
39	M	60	Left S3 PI (2–5)	30	2	2 h	0	Minimal	Nil	Yes
40	M	57	Left S3 PI (2–5)	30	2	2 h	0	Minimal	Nil	Yes

No.	Sex	Age	Procedure							
41	F	45	Right S3 PI (2–5)	40	4	2 ½ h	0	Minimal	Nil	Yes
42	F/C	12	Left ulnar nerve decompression	20–25	4	1 h	2	Moderate	Nil	Yes
43	M	30	Left S3 PI (2–5)	30	2	2 h	0	Minimal	Nil	Yes
44	M	35	Left PL PI (2–5)	60	4	3 h	2	Moderate	Nil	Yes
45	M	50	Left S3 PI (2–5) with ½ FPL to EPL	45	2	2 ½ h	0	Minimal	Nil	Yes
46	F	50	Right S3 PI (2–5) with ½ FPL to EPL	45	2	2 ½ h	0	Minimal	Nil	Yes
47	M	22	Left S3 PI (2–5) with ½ FPL to EPL	45	2	2 ½ h	0	Minimal	Nil	Yes
48	M	21	Right PL PI (2–5)	60	4	3 h	2	Moderate	Nil	Yes
49	M	15	Right PT to ECRB, FCR to EDC, & PL to EPL	45–50	4	3 h	2	Moderate	Nil	Yes
50	M	40	Right S3 PI (2–5)	30	2	2 h	0	Minimal	Nil	Yes
51	M	60	Right S4 to Thumb	30	2	1 ½ h	0	Minimal	Nil	Yes
52	M	27	Right S3 PI (2–5) with ½ FPL to EPL	45	4	2 ½ h	0	Minimal	Nil	Yes
53	M	40	Right S3 PI (2–5)	30	2	2 h	0	Moderate	Nil	Yes
54	M	60	Right S4 to Thumb	30	2	1 ½ h	0	Minimal	Nil	Yes
55	M	27	Right S3 PI (2–5) with ½ FPL to EPL	45	4	2 ½ h	0	Minimal	Nil	Yes
56	M	25	Right S3 PI (2–5)	30	2	2 h	0	Minimal	Nil	Yes

Ref	Abbreviation	Description
1	S3 PI (2–5)	Flexor digitorum sublimus of middle finger - 4 tail transfer to A1 pulley of fingers 2–4
	ECRL 4 T	ECRL extended with fascia lata - 4 tail transfer to A1 pulley of fingers 2–4
	PL PI (2–5)	PL extended with fascia lata - 4 tail transfer to A1 pulley of fingers 2–4
	S3 4T lateral band (2–5)	Flexor digitorum sublimus of middle finger - 4 tail transfer to lateral band of fingers 2–4
2	S3 PI (2–5) with 1/2 FPL to EPL	Flexor digitorum sublimus of middle finger - 4 tail transfer to A1 pulley of fingers 2–4 and one tail of flexor pollicis longus transferred to extensor pollicis longus
3	1/2 FPL to EPL	One tail of flexor pollicis longus transferred to extensor pollicis longus
4	S4 to thumb	Flexor digitorum sublimus of ring finger - 2 tail transfer to extensor pollicis longus & adductor of thumb
5	PT to ECRB, FCR to EDC, & PL to EPL	Pronator teres to ECRB, FCR to extensor digitorum communis, and PL transfer to extensor pollisis longus
6		Decompression of the nerve and debridement of the abscess
7		Full-thickness skin graft harvested from forearm or thigh applied after releasing contracture at PIP joint

Abbreviations: F, female; M, male.

incisions, the authors infiltrated 5 mL of solution at the MP joint of each finger. After half an hour, they moved the patient to the operating theater for surgery.

Comment from Dr Lalonde

I prefer to always inject my proximal incisions before my distal incisions. Proximal nerves become numb to decrease the pain of distal injections. As in the direct lasso procedure, I would inject the MP joints with only 2 injections between the metacarpal heads instead of 4 injections (one at each metacarpal head) (see earlier discussion).

Surgical Procedure

The following text describes what is seen in the images in **Fig. 7**.

Indirect lasso procedures are those in which a muscle other than FDS is used as the motor. PL or extensor carpi radialis longus (ECRL) are the muscles commonly used for motors. The tendon of the motor muscle is extended by means of fascia lata grafts.

First, the authors extracted a fascia lata graft 20 cm long and 1.5 cm wide from the anterolateral thigh under local anesthesia with a fascia stripper after they elevated the suprafascial tissue with a scissor though proximal and distal incisions (see **Fig. 7**A–D). The authors then made a 1- to 1.5-cm incision over the proximal volar crease at the wrist and detached the PL at its insertion (see **Fig. 7**E). The next incision was at the middle of the volar aspect of the forearm 5 cm above the proximal wrist crease, to deliver the PL tendon for ease of suturing of the fascia lata graft to the tendon (see **Fig. 7**F). The PL was lengthened by attaching a strip of fascia lata to it using the wrap-around technique of tendon repair (see **Fig. 7**G).

A 2-cm longitudinal incision was made just distal to the flexor retinaculum along the palm midline. The palmar aponeurosis was split, and the flexor synovial sheath was opened. The authors brought the tendon-graft assembly into the palm through the carpal tunnel with an Anderson tunneller (see **Fig. 7**H). They then split the fascia lata graft into 4 equal tails (see **Fig. 7**I).

As in the direct lasso procedure above, the authors made a curved incision connecting the radial end of middle palmar crease and the ulnar end of distal palmar crease. They developed flaps containing skin and subcutaneous fat distally up to the base of the fingers and proximally up to 1 cm to expose the A1 and A2 pulleys of each finger. They passed an Anderson tunneller or a curved artery forceps from the distal palmar incision through the radial interosseous space into the proximal longitudinal incision to pull each of the 4 tails through to each MP joint the palmar incision.

The authors took the tip of a tail with end of a mosquito forceps or a guide eye tunneler and passed it through the flexor tunnel to bring it out through middle of the A2 pulley. They then passed the other 3 tails through their respective flexor tunnels. They folded the tails back over the proximal half of A2 and A1 pulley in the right tension and fixed them to themselves proximal to the pulley with 2 or 3 sutures. The authors began with the little finger where they applied maximum tension with the MP joint at 90°. The authors decreased the MP angle in each finger by 10° as they went to the index finger to maintain the cascade.

The authors applied a short arm cast for 3 weeks to keep the wrist neutral, MP joints flexed, and interphalangeal joints extended.

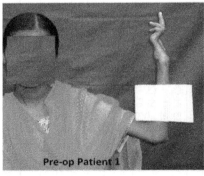
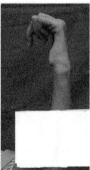
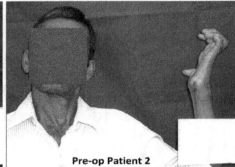

Fig. 2. Claw hand. Two preoperative patients who have 4 finger MP hyperextension resulting from ulnar nerve palsy from leprosy. They will be treated with the direct lasso procedure.

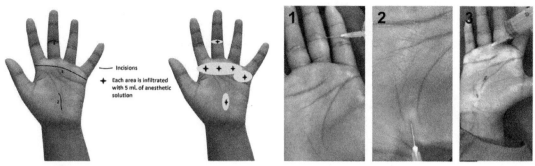

Fig. 3. Incisions and infiltration of anesthetic solution in claw hand deformity.

CORRECTION OF Z THUMB WITH HALF FLEXOR POLLICIS LONGUS TO EXTENSOR POLLICIS LONGUS

The z-thumb deformity results from ulnar nerve palsy. In ulnar nerve paralysis, the adductor pollicis, first dorsal interosseous, and often flexor pollicis brevis are paralyzed. Loss of adductor pollicis causes marked weakening of key pinch. Loss of flexor pollicis brevis causes hyperflexion of the interphalangeal joint, and/or hyperextension of the MP joint. For a Z thumb deformity, half flexor pollicis longus (FPL) to extensor pollicis longus (EPL) transfer gives a good result, especially for isolated interphalangeal joint hyperflexion.

LOCAL ANESTHETIC TECHNIQUE

The images of the local anesthetic injection sites in **Fig. 8** are those of a normal thumb, not a Z thumb. For Z-thumb correction, 3 to 5 mL of prepared solution was infiltrated in the flexion crease in the interphalangeal joint of thumb until visible, and palpable local anesthesia was seen in dissection areas. In a similar fashion, 3 to 5 mL of solution was infiltrated in the proximal volar crease of the MP joint. For the third incision, 5 mL of solution was infiltrated in the middle of the dorsal aspect of the proximal phalanx.

Comment from Dr Lalonde

I prefer to inject in the subcutaneous fat in the middle of the volar and dorsal thumb and finger phalanges, instead of in the creases. I have found that injections into my own thumb and finger creases are more painful than in the noncrease tissues. Injecting in the midline of the palmar aspect of digits just under the skin avoids the needle poking one of the digital nerves, which is unnecessarily painful and could injure the nerve.

SURGICAL PROCEDURE

The following text describes what is seen in the images in **Fig. 9**.

The authors made a 1- to 1.5-cm incision over the volar crease of the interphalangeal joint of the thumb. They then identified the radial half of FPL (see **Fig. 9**A) and split the tendon to the level of the MP joint (see **Fig. 9**B). The authors then detached the radial half of FPL from its insertion (see **Fig. 9**C). They made a second 1.5-cm incision in the proximal volar crease of the thumb MP joint and FPL was identified (see **Fig. 9**D). Then the separated radial slip of the FPL was retracted outside the incision.

The authors made a third 2-cm oblique incision over the dorsal surface of proximal phalanx of thumb to identify EPL (see **Fig. 9**E). They then passed an Anderson tunneller or curved mosquito forceps from the dorsal incision into the proximal volar incision to pull FPL through the dorsal incision. The authors sutured FPL to the EPL, keeping the thumb in 20° flexion at MP and interphalangeal joint by 2 to 3 sutures (see **Fig. 9**F). **Fig. 9**G demonstrates the thumb showing the desired position after the procedure.

Comment from Dr Lalonde

At this point, I would get the patient to flex and extend the thumb to test the tension of the tendon transfer and make sure it is correct. I could adjust or reinforce my sutures if necessary, before closing the skin.

The authors then closed the dorsal incision and immobilized the thumb for 3 weeks using a forearm back slab and a thumb slab to hold the thumb in abduction at carpometacarpal joint, 30° flexion at the MP joint, and the interphalangeal joint straight.

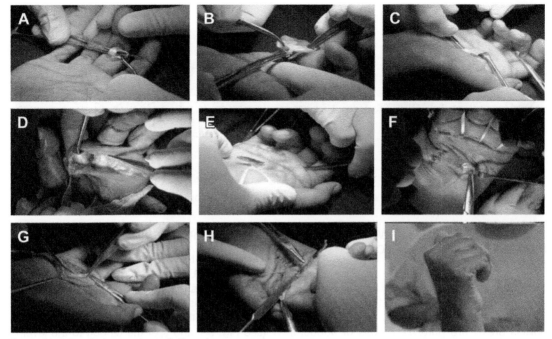

Fig. 4. (*A–I*) Surgical procedure of direct lasso procedure.

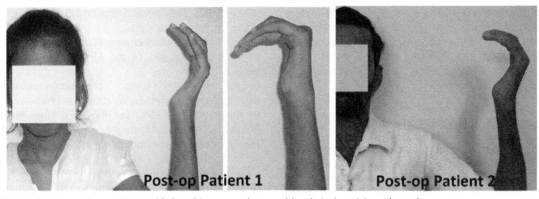

Post-op Patient 1   Post-op Patient 2

Fig. 5. Postoperative patients with hand in open ulnar and lumbrical position ulnar view.

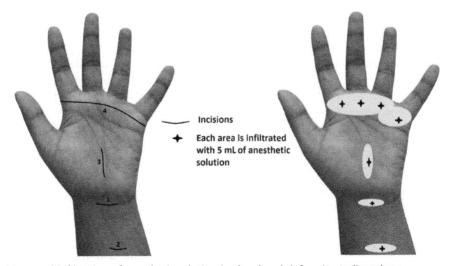

Incisions

Each area is infiltrated with 5 mL of anesthetic solution

Fig. 6. Incisions and infiltration of anesthetic solution in claw hand deformity. Indirect lasso.

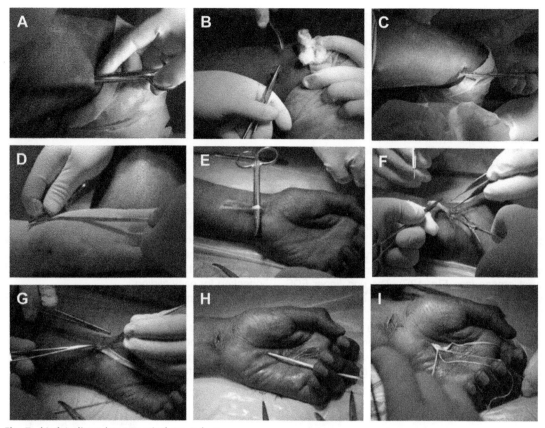

Fig. 7. (A–I) Indirect lasso surgical procedure.

RESTORATION OF THUMB ABDUCTION/ OPPOSITION WITH OPPONENSPLASTY: SUPERFICIALIS TRANSFER WITH DOUBLE INSERTION TECHNIQUE

In pure median nerve palsy, MP flexion of the thumb is preserved, and adduction/opposition is the goal of the tendon transfer (**Fig. 10**).

LOCAL ANESTHETIC TECHNIQUE

The images of the local anesthetic injection sites in **Fig. 11** are those of a normal thumb, not a paralyzed thumb. The authors started with 5 mL of prepared solution in the proximal flexion crease in the PIP joint of the ring finger. For the second incision, 5 mL of prepared solution was infiltrated 3 cm proximal to the distal wrist crease over the forearm. For the third incision, the authors infiltrated 5 mL at the area distal and radial to the pisiform. For the fourth incision, 5 mL was infiltrated at mid palm point of the thumb MP joint. For the fifth incision, 5 mL of prepared solution was infiltrated over the radial/dorsal side of the MP joint of thumb. Finally, 5 mL of solution was infiltrated

distal of the dorsal proximal phalanx and another 5 mL in the basal joint area (for incisions 5 and 6).

> **Comment from Dr Lalonde**
>
> The 35 mL of local anesthesia seems small for the large areas of tunneling required in this operation. All tunnels must be numb with at least 2 cm of visible and palpable local anesthesia on either side of the tunnels. It is better to err on the side of too much local anesthesia instead of not enough local anesthesia. You can decrease the concentration to 0.5% lidocaine with 1:200,000 epinephrine to have 100 mL available and keep within safe limits of lidocaine in larger hands. The goal is a pain-free patient experience with no "top ups" of extra intraoperative injections of local anesthesia.

SURGICAL PROCEDURE

The following text describes what is seen in the images in **Fig. 12**.

The authors made a 1- to 1.5-cm in the volar crease of the PIP joint of the ring finger. The

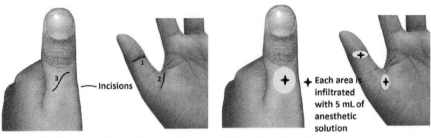

Fig. 8. Incisions and infiltration of anesthetic solution in Z-thumb deformity.

authors identified FDP and retracted it radially and ulnarly to detach the 2 slips of FDS from their insertion (see **Fig. 12**A). They separated the 2 slips at their chiasm.

The authors then made a second 1.5 cm transverse incision about 3 cm proximal to the distal wrist crease (see **Fig. 12**B). The ring finger FDS was identified and brought out of this incision (see **Fig. 12**C).

A third 8-mm incision was made 1 cm distal and radial to the pisiform and deepened until the loose large fat lobules of Guyon canal were seen protruding up from the small firm fat globules typical

of the palm. A small curved Anderson tunneller was then passed from the pisiform incision to the forearm incision, passing deep to the pisohamate ligament and emerging in the same plane as the ulnar nerve and artery (see **Fig. 12**D). The tendon was then withdrawn into the palm and checked for easy gliding.

A fourth 1-cm incision was made palmar to the MP joint. With the Anderson tunneller, the FDS tendon was then passed deep subcutaneously into the thumb MP incision and again checked for free gliding (see **Fig. 12**E). Both the slips were then widely separated up to 5 cm proximally (see **Fig. 12**F).

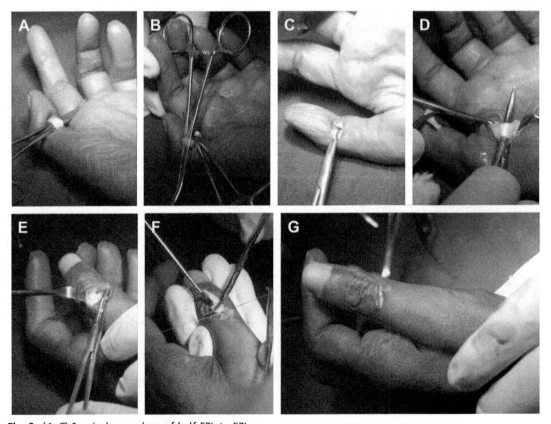

Fig. 9. (A–G) Surgical procedure of half FPL to EPL.

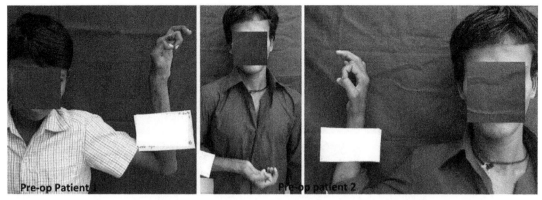

Fig. 10. Lack of abduction/opposition deformity in 2 preoperative patients resulting from median nerve palsy. They will be treated with Brand's procedure.

A fifth 1.5-cm curved incision was made over the insertion of the adductor pollicis and a sixth oblique 2-cm incision was made over the dorsal surface of proximal phalanx of thumb. The authors identified EPL (see **Fig. 12**G). One FDS slip was passed just distal to the MP joint over the dorsal aspect and then looped around the adductor insertion adjacent to bone (see **Fig. 12**H). It is important to keep this slip distal to the MP to prevent a Z-thumb deformity. The other slip is routed palmar to the MP joint to insert with a triple weave on EPL (see **Fig. 12**I). This insertion on EPL serves as an MP flexor as well as IP extensor to correct the deformity arising from the FPB paralysis. All the incisions are sutured.

Comment from Dr Lalonde

At this point, I would get the patient to flex and extend the thumb to test the tension of the tendon transfer and make sure it is correct. I could adjust or reinforce my sutures if necessary, before closing the skin.

The hand is immobilized with the wrist flexed 15° to 20° and the thumb in full opposition and abduction for 3 weeks (**Fig. 13**).

Tendon Transfers for Radial Nerve Palsy

The authors usually transfer pronator teres (PT) to extensor carpi radialis brevis (ECRB), flexor carpi radialis (FCR) to extensor digitorum communis (EDC) and PL to EPL.

LOCAL ANESTHETIC TECHNIQUE

The images of the local anesthetic injection sites in **Fig. 14** are those of a normal hand, not a hand with radial nerve palsy.

For wrist drop correction (**Fig. 15**), 15 mL of prepared solution was infiltrated over the middle of the lateral aspect of the semipronated forearm including deep to the muscle and touching the bone. For the second incision, 5 mL of prepared solution was infiltrated around the volar aspect of middle of the proximal wrist crease. For the third incision, 10 mL of prepared solution was infiltrated

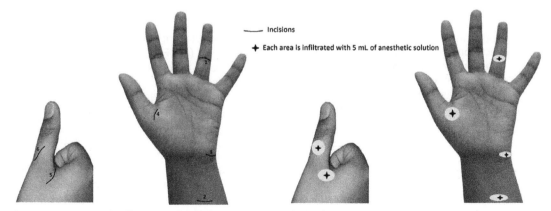

— Incisions

✛ Each area is infiltrated with 5 mL of anesthetic solution

Fig. 11. Incisions and infiltration of anesthetic solution in lack of adduction/opposition.

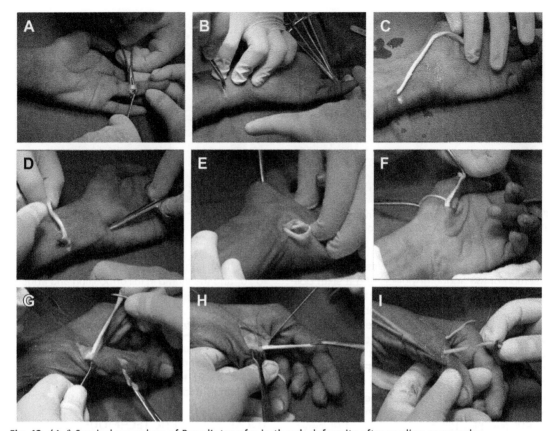

Fig. 12. (*A–I*) Surgical procedure of Brand's transfer in thumb deformity after median nerve palsy.

longitudinally 5 cm proximal to the wrist crease. For the fourth incision, 10 mL of prepared solution was infiltrated at middle of the dorsum of the wrist. For the fifth incision, 5 mL of prepared solution was infiltrated proximal to Lister tubercle. For the sixth incision, 3 mL of prepared solution was infiltrated over the area proximal to the MP joint of the thumb.

Comment from Dr Lalonde

For this transfer, I would usually use 100 to 200 mL of 0.25% lidocaine with 1:400,000 epinephrine buffered with bicarbonate to which I add 20 mL of bupivacaine with epinephrine. I inject from proximal to distal. I would like visible or palpable local anesthetic 2 cm beyond anywhere I am going to dissect or make tunnels through tissue. The goal is to not hurt the patient at all during surgery, and to not require "top ups" of painful extra local anesthetic injection during the surgery.

SURGICAL PROCEDURE

The following text describes what is seen in the images in **Fig. 16**.

An 8- to 10-cm curved incision is made over the convex part of the middle of the radial border of the forearm to expose the insertion of the PT and the ECRB tendon. The tendons are encircled with a towel clip (see **Fig. 16**A). At this level, the ECRB tendon is usually surrounded by muscle, but the tendon is easily found inside. The insertion of PT is identified by following the muscle down to its fanlike insertion on the radius. It is detached with its periosteum from the lateral border of radius (see **Fig. 16**B).

A longitudinal incision is made on the midpoint of the dorsum of the wrist, and the extensor retinaculum is cut along the same line to expose the 4 slips of EDC (see **Fig. 16**C). A transverse incision is then made over the volar aspect of proximal wrist crease, and tendons of PL and FCR are identified; both are detached at their insertions. A 4-cm curved incision is made 5 cm proximal to wrist crease where both the tendons of PL and FCR are brought out of this incision (see **Fig. 16**D).

Through a longitudinal incision just proximal to Lister tubercle over the level of the extensor retinaculum, the EPL is identified and isolated. It is divided at its musculotendinous junction. This tendon is withdrawn distally, through an incision

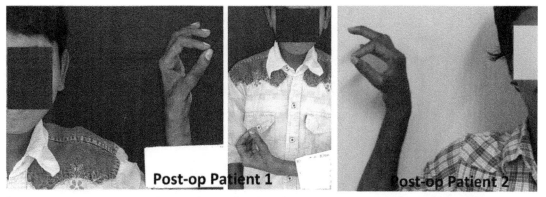

Fig. 13. Postoperative patients showing better thumb adduction/opposition for index thumb pinch.

just proximal to the MP joint of the thumb (see **Fig. 16**E). It is tunneled subcutaneously to over the proximal incision in the volar forearm beside the tendon of PL.

The PT is then brought around, superficial to the brachioradialis, to avoid adhesions to the radius. The PT is passed through the ECRB tendon as far distally as possible and sutured with braided nylon with moderate (1 cm) tension. The end is buried in the muscle, and the repair is covered with 6-0 monofilament nylon (see **Fig. 16**F).

The FCR is tunneled subcutaneously into this incision, finding the path of least resistance using a blunt instrument. With the wrist in about 45° extension, and the fingers extended fully at the MP joints, the FCR tendon is passed through the individual slips of the EDC as distally as possible after taking up the slack. It is sutured in such a manner as to incorporate all the tendons in the stitch (see **Fig. 16**G). The PL and EPL tendons are sutured with a short interlace, under high tension, with the thumb positioned in extension in the same plane as the palm (see **Fig. 16**H).

Comment from Dr Lalonde

At this point, I would get the patient to flex and extend the thumb, fingers, and wrist to test the tension of the tendon transfers and make sure it is correct. I could adjust or reinforce my sutures if necessary, before closing the skin.

The skin incisions are then closed. The wrist is immobilized in 45° of extension for 3 weeks before mobilization is commenced (see **Fig. 16**I; **Fig. 17**).

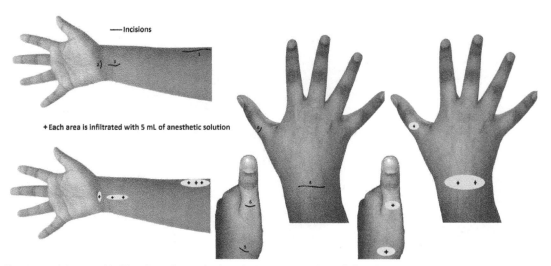

Fig. 14. Incisions and infiltration of anesthetic solution in wrist drop deformity.

82   Mohammed & Lalonde

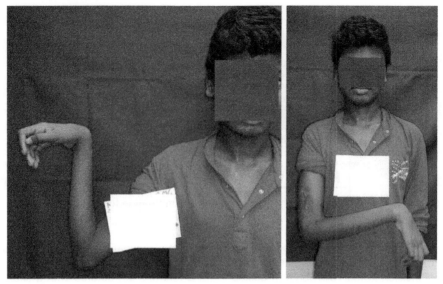

Fig. 15. Wrist drop deformity in preoperative patient resulting from radial nerve palsy from leprosy. There is a scar in anterolateral arm due to incision and drainage of a radial nerve abscess that occurred as a result of leprosy.

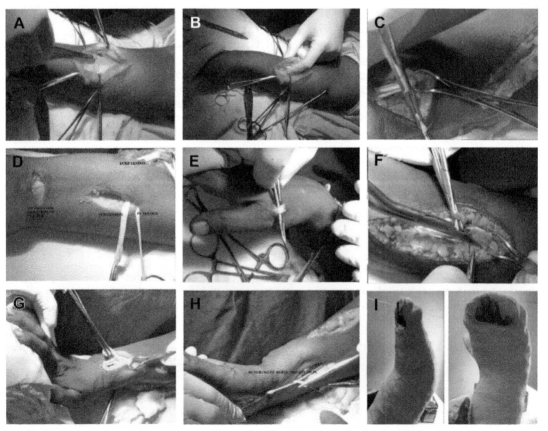

Fig. 16. (*A–I*) Surgical procedure to restore finger, thumb, and wrist extension in radial nerve palsy.

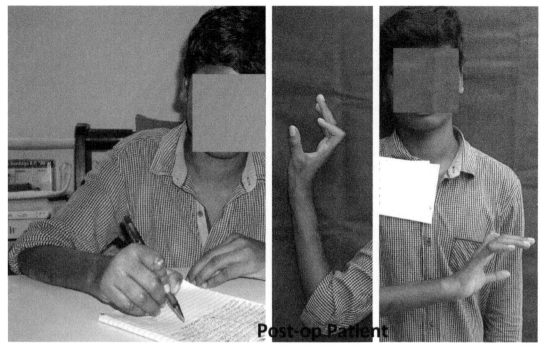

Fig. 17. Postoperative patient writing and extending wrist and fingers.

SUMMARY: THE EARLY NELLORE IMPRESSIONS OF WIDE AWAKE LOCAL ANESTHESIA NO TOURNIQUET TENDON TRANSFERS IN LEPROSY PATIENTS

The WALANT technique offers effective anesthetic and hemostatic effects with an almost painless and bloodless operative field in tendon transfers for leprosy. The amount of solution injected ranged from 20 to 45 mL, with an additional 30 mL for infiltration of tumescent local anesthesia into anterolateral thigh for extraction of fascia lata graft. Tendon tensioning was more effective when the patient was awake. No patient expressed significant pain while they were injected with tumescent local anesthesia and while they had the surgery. Most of the procedures took approximately 2 hours' time.

Before WALANT, the authors used axillary blocks and the tourniquet. It was great to be able to eliminate tourniquet pain that patients frequently had to tolerate. The authors also were pleased to eliminate some of the difficulties they had with axillary blocks.

There was minimal bleeding in some of the cases, which was overcome by compression and by pressure. This is in line with experience in tendon transfer for other hand disorders or primary repairs.[7–11] Blood loss was decreased because there was no let down bleeding effect with the elimination of the tourniquet.

All the patients were comfortable with WALANT. They all have requested this technique for their future surgeries because they have had bilateral deformities because of multiple nerve palsies due to leprosy.

This disease is prevalent in more disadvantaged social-economic groups. The Damien foundation is a voluntary organization where cost-effectiveness plays an important role. The WALANT technique helped to cut expenses of the procedures as the authors eliminated the cost of anesthesiologists, their equipment, and their medications. That money has been invested to perform more surgeries.

As surgeons, the authors appreciated the fact that there were no anesthetic inconveniences or complications to deal with before, during, and after the surgery. Patients liked and appreciated the opportunity to have surgery this way.

The authors conclude that WALANT with tumescent local anesthesia in reconstructive surgeries in hand in leprosy offers is an effective low-cost technique.

REFERENCES

1. Donald Lalonde MD, Alison Martin MD. Epinephrine in local anesthesia in finger and hand surgery: the case for wide-awake anesthesia. J Am Acad Orthop Surg 2013;21:443–7.

2. Klein JA. Tumescent technique for regional anesthesia permits lidocaine doses of 35 mg/kg for liposuction. J Dermatol Surg Oncol 1990;16:248–63.
3. Bieniek A, Orzechowska-Juzwenko K, Gowacka K, et al. Tumescent local anesthesia (TLA) and its practical signification in modern surgery (Polish). Wrocaw (Poland): MedPharm; 2007.
4. Prasetyono TO. Tourniquet-free hand surgery using the one-per-mil tumescent technique. Arch Plast Surg 2013;40:129–33.
5. Lalonde DH. "Hole-in-one" local anesthesia for wide-awake carpal tunnel surgery. Plast Reconstr Surg 2010;126:1642–4.
6. Lalonde D. How the wide awake approach is changing hand surgery and hand therapy: inaugural AAHS sponsored lecture at the ASHT meeting, San Diego, 2012. J Hand Ther 2013;26:175–8.
7. Lalonde DH. Conceptual origins, current practice, and views of wide awake hand surgery. J Hand Surg Eur 2017;42:886–95.
8. Xing SG, Mao T. Temporary tourniquet use after epinephrine injection to expedite wide awake emergency hand surgeries. J Hand Surg Eur 2018;43:888–9.
9. Lalonde DH, Kozin S. Tendon disorders of the hand. Plast Reconstr Surg 2011;128:1e–14e.
10. Lalonde DH. Wide-awake extensor indicis proprius to extensor pollicis longus tendon transfer. J Hand Surg Am 2014;39:2297–9.
11. Bezuhly M, Sparkes GL, Higgins A, et al. Immediate thumb extension following extensor indicis proprius-to-extensor pollicis longus tendon transfer using the wide-awake approach. Plast Reconstr Surg 2007;15;119:1507–12.

Wide-Awake Wrist and Small Joints Arthroscopy of the Hand

Bo Liu, MD, FRCS[a],*, Chye Yew Ng, FRCS, DipHandSurg (Br&Eur)[b],
Mohammed Shoaib Arshad, MBChB, FRCS[b],
Dafydd S. Edwards, FRCS, MD[b],
Michael J. Hayton, MBChB, FRCS[b]

KEYWORDS

• Anesthesia • Wide-awake hand surgery • Wrist arthroscopy • Small joint arthroscopy • WALANT

KEY POINTS

• The minimally invasive nature of wrist and small joint arthroscopy renders it particularly suitable for the application of the wide-awake local anesthesia no tourniquet (WALANT) technique.
• During arthroscopy of the small joints in the hand, the surgeon is able to show and discuss with the patient the pathology identified and its management while viewing the internal architecture of the joint. For some patients, the ability to visualize their repaired or débrided structures reinforces their confidence in the surgeon and encourages them to comply with postoperative rehabilitation.
• The extended application of dynamic wide-awake wrist arthroscopy has provided new insight in the assessment of carpal instability and has also challenged current understanding of carpal kinetics.
• With increased familiarity with WALANT, the spectrum of procedures that can be safely performed inside small joints using wide-awake technique is expected to rise.

INTRODUCTION

Compared with open procedures of the hand, application of wide-awake local anesthesia no tourniquet (WALANT) technique in small joint and wrist arthroscopies is still limited, with only a few published series.[1–4] The minimally invasive nature of arthroscopy renders it particularly suitable for WALANT technique. In addition, the option of intra-articular fluid irrigation and distention allows for control of internal bleeding, should it become necessary. During arthroscopy, the surgeon is able to show and discuss with the patient the pathology identified and its management while viewing the internal architecture of the joint. For some patients, the ability to visualize their repaired or débrided structures reinforces their confidence in the surgeon and encourages them to comply with postoperative rehabilitation. This article reports experience in 2 centers on the application of WALANT technique in arthroscopy of the wrist and small joints of the hand.

Between 2012 and 2017, the author (BL) at Beijing Ji Shui Tan Hospital (Beijing) performed 31 wide-awake arthroscopies (22 wrists and 9 small joints of the hand). Between 2016 and 2018, the authors (MH, CN) at Wrightington Hospital (Wigan) performed 20 dynamic wide-awake wrist arthroscopies (d-WAWAs). The range of procedures is summarized in **Table 1**. The authors' techniques are summarized.

Disclosure Statement: The authors have nothing to disclose.
[a] Department of Hand Surgery, Beijing Ji Shui Tan Hospital, 4th Clinical Hospital of Peking University, 31 Xinjiekou East Street, Beijing 100035, China; [b] Upper Limb Unit, Wrightington Hospital, Hall Lane, Appley Bridge, Wigan, Lancashire WN6 9EP, UK
* Corresponding author.
E-mail address: bobliu7@hotmail.com

Hand Clin 35 (2019) 85–92
https://doi.org/10.1016/j.hcl.2018.08.010

Table 1
Range of procedures and number of patients who underwent wide-awake wrist and small joint arthroscopies in two units

Arthroscopy	Surgical Procedures	Number of Patients
Wrist arthroscopy	Exploration	7
	Synovectomy	6
	Dorsal wrist ganglionectomy	3
	TFCC débridement	5
	TFCC repair	1
Dynamic wrist arthroscopy	Diagnostic	20
Carpometacarpal joint arthroscopy	Loose body removal	2
	Synovectomy	3
	Thermal shrinkage	1
MCP joint arthroscopy	Synovectomy	2
PIP joint arthroscopy	Synovectomy	1

PORTAL SITE LOCAL ANESTHESIA

The key for a successful wide-awake arthroscopy is effective portal site local anesthesia.[4] This demands a sound appreciation of surface anatomy and precise technique in creating an arthroscopy portal. To prevent secondary movement of the skin, the authors recommend that the limb is secured with the necessary traction before infiltrating local anesthetic. In comparison to open WALANT procedures, where a generous volume of local anesthetic and substantial waiting time are generally recommended, only a small volume of local anesthetic and minimal waiting time are required for effective portal site local anesthesia. For those patients on anticoagulants, the use of adrenaline in the portal sites also allows this technique to be used in patients with an international normalized ratio of up to 3.

There are some technical tips when performing portal site local anesthesia for wrist arthroscopy. The authors prefer using 1% lignocaine with 1:200,000 adrenaline using a 27-gauge needle. Once the skin bleb is created, the needle is advanced toward the capsule. While the needle is advanced, local anesthetic is injected slowly along its path of entrance. Once the resistance of wrist capsule is felt, local anesthetic is injected slightly more quickly due to the increased amount of nerve fibers in the capsule. Finally, once the capsule is breached, the needle is withdrawn slowly and local anesthetic infiltrated again along its path of withdrawal. Generally, 2 mL of local anesthetic is sufficient for anesthetizing a single portal site. If intra-articular therapeutic maneuver, such as synovectomy or débridement, is indicated, then an additional 4 mL of intra-articular local anesthetic should afford adequate anesthesia (**Fig. 1**).

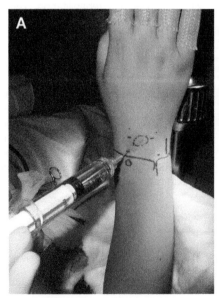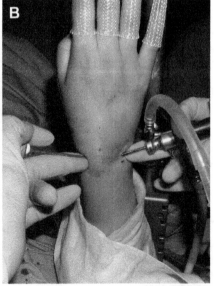

Fig. 1. (*A*) Portal site local anesthesia before creation of wrist arthroscopy portals in a patient who underwent arthroscopic ganglionectomy. (*B*) WALANT arthroscopic ganglionectomy was performed immediately after portal site local anesthesia.

The portal site local anesthesia and open WALANT infiltration techniques can also be combined. For instance, after diagnostic wrist arthroscopy under portal site local anesthesia, an open triangular fibrocartilage complex (TFCC) repair was required in 1 of the authors' patients. The open repair was well tolerated and successfully performed using an additional 10 mL of local anesthetic injected slowly around the distal ulnar region, as per original tumescent local anesthesia WALANT technique.

WIDE-AWAKE WRIST ARTHROSCOPY

The setup of wide-awake wrist arthroscopy is essentially the same as when it is performed under general or regional anesthesia. The patient is placed supine with the shoulder abducted and elbow flexed. The wrist is suspended using an arthroscopy tower, according to surgeon preference. It is important to achieve sufficient and tolerable traction to ensure ease of portal creation and comfort of the patient during the wide-awake procedure. The standard portals of 3/4, 4/5, 6R, 6U, MCR, and MCU can be established.

One unique feature of wide-awake arthroscopy compared with open WALANT procedures is the ready availability of the screen visualization of the condition of the joint and ongoing reconstruction, which can be viewed continuously and simultaneously by the patient and surgeon. For the open procedures, a direct viewing of the wound by the patient is still possible, but this can add time to the procedure.

During arthroscopic portal establishment, dorsal synovectomy, dorsal wrist ganglion excision, and TFCC repair, the extensor tendons are at risk of being damaged. Although the application of WALANT technique has not eliminated the risks completely, it does allow immediate assessment of finger movements and integrity of the moving extensor tendons intraoperatively. Any injury can thus be visualized more easily and addressed promptly.

DYNAMIC WIDE-AWAKE WRIST ARTHROSCOPY—WRIGHTINGTON EXPERIENCE

With increasing experience in wide-awake wrist arthroscopy, there has been further advancement of the application. Traditionally wrist arthroscopy has been a passive, nondynamic investigation. The published series of wide-awake wrist arthroscopy thus far, however, have not incorporated the intraoperative dynamic element that this procedure offers. The authors describe a d-WAWA that allows the patient to grip and release with the wrist

arthroscope in situ. With this technique, the in vivo carpal kinetics can be observed and assessed in a more realistic manner than previously possible.

The main clinical indication for d-WAWA, over and above nondynamic wrist arthroscopy, is in the assessment of carpal instability. The diagnosis of instability has been traditionally made on the grounds of observing abnormal spacing between the various bones by using a probe inside the wrist. Assessment of scapholunate instability is performed using the Geissler classification in a nondynamic setting.[5] The original description uses a 3-mm probe to try to assess any gaps between the scaphoid and lunate with the patient asleep. In contrast, the gapping can still be assessed with a probe in d-WAWA and then further assessed with even better visualization during, active patient movement in the dynamic phase of the procedure.

Preoperative and Intraoperative Preparation

Preoperative selection of suitable patients is particularly important for the success of the procedure. The patient needs to be compliant and willing to engage actively during the procedure. The authors' main reservation for this procedure is an uncooperative or nervous patient. It is, therefore, important in the outpatient clinic to carefully assess the personality of the patient to ensure that they would be suitable for d-WAWA. Another relative contraindication is in a wrist that has heavy scarring from previous surgery or injury, which makes portal creation and intra-articular maneuvering challenging.

There are some important modifications to that of conventional wrist arthroscopy. The main variation is the method by which the arm is suspended for the procedure. Classic finger traps cannot be used for d-WAWA, because the patient is unable to grip when requested. The authors have developed a specific hand holder (using a chinstrap used by the anesthetists) that suspends the hand and allows active gripping. (A commercially available holder is being developed and will be suitable for either d-WAWA or conventional wrist arthroscopy.) The patient is positioned supine and a chinstrap is suspended from a typical arthroscopy tower next to the patient above an arm board. The patient is asked to grip the chinstrap (**Fig. 2**A), which is then secured to the hand using broad adhesive draping tape to prevent the hand from losing grip and falling down when the patient relaxes the grip (**Fig. 2**B). The chinstrap can be attached above and distally to a standard arthroscopy suspension pole (**Fig. 3**). Once the hand is secure, the authors recommend a series of rehearsed grip maneuvers to be performed by

A   **B**

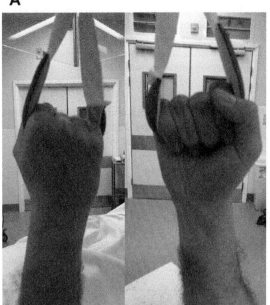
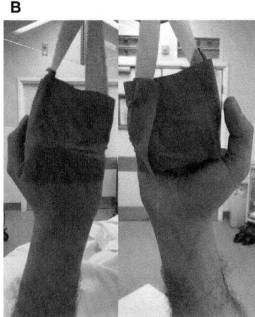

Fig. 2. The novel method of holding the hand allows dynamic gripping during the procedure that would otherwise not be possible using standard finger traps. (*A*) The hand is gripping the strap ensuring ability to make a fist. (*B*) The hand is then secured with sticky tape.

the patient. Such maneuvers are grip, ulnar deviation, and radial deviation. The authors have found that this practice is invaluable and allows patients to understand what is expected of them in the

dynamic phase of the procedure. The authors do not usually use weighted countertraction of the arm for d-WAWA. The weight of the arm is usually sufficient to distract the joint. Besides, excessive external distraction may mask subtle instability by virtue of ligamentotaxis.

Only when a patient is well positioned and the arm is suspended are skin markings of the portals and local anesthetic infiltration performed to prevent secondary movement of the skin relative to the underlying wrist joint. The timing of local anesthetic infiltration has also been modified. Prior to formal draping, but under aseptic technique, portal sites are injected with local anesthetic. The authors suggest waiting several minutes for the local anesthetic to be effective (**Fig. 4**). Once the skin has been anesthetized and the effect of adrenaline causing local vasoconstriction is seen, the surgeon is then able to scrub. Once gowned, the surgeon returns to the arm, preps and drapes the arm in a routine fashion. Further local anesthetic is then injected down to the dorsal aspect of the wrist capsule with plain 0.25% bupivacaine. The joint is then infiltrated with local anesthetic, although in some patients a dry arthroscopy is possible without causing discomfort.

Dynamic Assessment

First, a standard assessment of the radiocarpal and midcarpal joints is performed. Next, the intercarpal spaces are probed in a routine manner. Should there

Fig. 3. The chinstrap can be attached above and distally to a standard arthroscopy suspension pole.

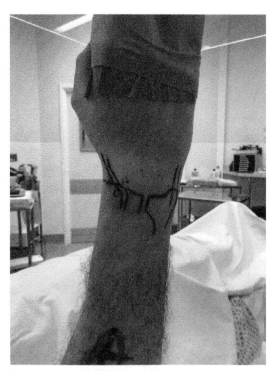

Fig. 4. Vasoconstriction achieved using adrenaline combined with the local anesthetic.

be any laxity, such as in the scapholunate interval, the gapping is then assessed in a dynamic manner by asking the patient to make a fist and then relax. It is of utmost importance that when assessing dynamic instability with the patient gripping, the arthroscope is held just inside the dorsal wrist capsule and not deep inside the joint. Compressive forces that occur when the hand grips may cause damage to the articular cartilage and arthroscope.

The authors have observed on several occasions, in patients with a positive drive-through sign of scapholunate interval (grade 4 tear), that the gap between scaphoid and lunate closes on gripping rather than the classic teaching that the gap would widen further. This phenomenon has not been described previously and requires further evaluation, discussion of which is beyond the scope of this article. Apart from carpal instability, d-WAWA also has the utility in assessing distal radioulnar joint instability that help informs appropriate treatment of a TFCC lesion.

Complications

The authors have not found this d-WAWA technique to have increased the surgical risks over and above conventional wrist arthroscopy. The authors recognize the potential risk of damaging the cartilage and the arthroscope during gripping

maneuvers but this may be avoided by having sound arthroscopic skills.

WIDE-AWAKE SMALL JOINT ARTHROSCOPY OF THE HAND

The setup for wide-awake arthroscopy for the small joints of the hand is essentially the same as that when the procedure is performed under general or regional anesthesia. Suspension and traction of the limb are necessary when performing arthroscopy of the thumb carpometacarpal joint and metacarpophalangeal (MCP) joint. In contrast, the hand can be simply placed on table for finger proximal interphalangeal (PIP) joint arthroscopy.

Thumb Carpometacarpal Joint Arthroscopy

The thumb is placed on 3kg to 5kg of longitudinal traction to facilitate joint distraction. The standard portals are on either side of the abductor pollicis longus (APL)/extensor pollicis brevis (EPB), namely 1R and 1U.[6] Accessory portals, such as the thenar portal[7] and the dorsal-distal (D2) portal,[8] have been described for specific circumstances. Regardless of the portal used, the technique of portal site local anesthesia and subsequent establishment of portal need to be precise and accurate to avoid undue discomfort to the patient. Intra-articular infiltration of local anesthetic is optional depending on the therapeutic maneuver indicated (**Fig. 5**). The authors prefer using a 1.9-mm arthroscope with a 30° viewing angle.

Metacarpophalangeal Joint Arthroscopy

The finger or thumb is placed on a digital trap/tube, which is then suspended on an arthroscopy tower. The joint space is easily appreciable by observing the skin dimples when the digit is under axial traction. The portals for thumb MCP joint arthroscopy are 1R and 1U, which are on either side of the extensor pollicis longus (EPL)/extensor pollicis brevis (EPB) tendons. Portal site local anesthesia is performed as described initially and fluid irrigation is used if necessary (**Fig. 6**).

Proximal Interphalangeal Joint Arthroscopy

When performing PIP joint arthroscopy, the hand is placed on top of a rolled-up towel. The standard portals are PIP-R and PIP-U (**Fig. 7**). Either portal can be established first depending on the condition of the finger and surgeon preference. After portal site local anesthesia, axial traction applied by an assistant would help to distract the joint while an 18-gauge needle is introduced into the joint, just palmar to the lateral band. A stab incision of 0.5 cm is made over the entry point before blunt

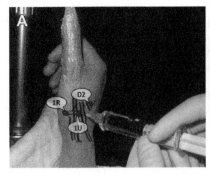
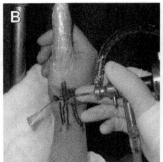
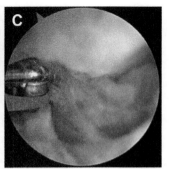

Fig. 5. (A) Portal site local anesthesia before creation of the portals of thumb carpometacarpal joint arthroscopy in a patient who underwent arthroscopic synovectomy. (B, C) WALANT arthroscopic synovectomy was performed immediately after portal site local anesthesia.

dissection using a mosquito clip to gain access of the joint. The authors prefer using a 1.9-mm diameter scope with a 30° viewing angle. The PIP-R and PIP-U portals are interchangeable for viewing and instrumentation. Generally, for diagnostic arthroscopy, intra-articular infiltration of local anesthetic is not necessary, but it can be added if synovectomy or débridement is planned. Fluid irrigation, if required, is by gravity alone.

Results

The portal site local anesthesia was well tolerated by all patients, with the reported visual analog scale (VAS) score for pain being less than 3. Among the patients who underwent wrist arthroscopy, only 1 of the 6 patients who needed synovectomy complained of slight pain (VAS score <3) during the procedure. Before ganglionectomy in 3 patients, 4 mL of local anesthesia was injected intra-articularly and the procedure was carried out successfully without noticeable pain. Of the 9 patients who underwent small joint arthroscopy, only 2 complained of slight pain (VAS score <3) during the procedures

(synovectomy and thermal shrinkage). The rest proceeded without noticeable pain.

PAST REPORTS FROM OTHER UNITS

Ho and colleagues[1] published the report of 5 patients undergoing volar ganglionectomies via standard wrist arthroscopy under local anesthesia. They reported no complications in their series. Hagert and Lalonde[3] presented 9 patients requiring wide-awake wrist arthroscopy for indications, such as interosseous ligament injuries, midcarpal instabilities, ulnotriquetral and TFCC tears, loose articular bodies, and arthroscopic release of wrist contracture. Their main contraindication was poor peripheral circulation. They used 20 mL of 1% lidocaine with epinephrine and 2 mL sodium bicarbonate; 5 mL lidocaine with epinephrine was injected intra-articularly and they waited 30 minutes to 50 minutes before starting the procedure to allow time for the anesthetic to work. Their setup included having the patient supine with the shoulder abducted at 90°, elbow flexed at 90°, forearm pronated, and the hand elevated using finger traps

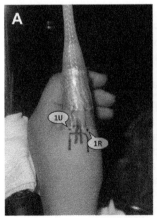
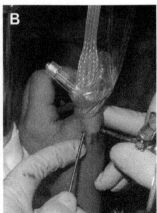
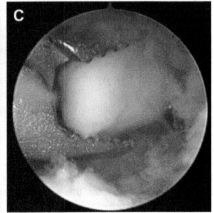

Fig. 6. (A) Portals for thumb MCP joint arthroscopy. (B, C) WALANT arthroscopic removal of loose body was performed immediately after portal site local anesthesia.

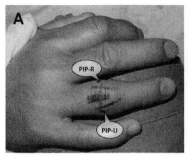
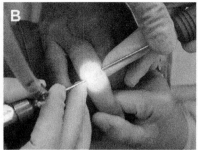
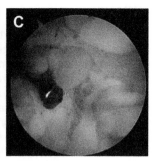

Fig. 7. (A) Portals for ring finger PIP joint arthroscopy in a patient with rheumatoid arthritis. (B, C) WALANT arthroscopic PIP joint synovectomy was performed immediately after portal site local anesthesia.

and a traction tower (with a traction force of 5kg). No tourniquet was used. Standard dorsal and midcarpal portals were used and again apart from mild pain (average VAS score 0–1) there were no significant complications.

Koo and Ho[9] presented a summary of their technique but alluded to their previous study on 111 patients.[2] Their indications for performing wrist arthroscopy under portal site local anesthetic included arthroscopic débridement, removal of loose body, synovectomy and biopsy, ganglionectomy, TFCC injuries, thermal shrinkage for interosseous ligament, release of wrist contracture, radial styloidectomy, arthroscopic wafer procedure, distal scaphoidectomy, chronic wrist pain of uncertain origin, and infective and carpal instability. Contraindications included hypersensitivity to lidocaine and epinephrine; cardiac disease (relative); procedures that required extensive bone work; and patient factors, such as young/immature and mental illness. Both articles described using 1% or 2% lidocaine with 1:200,000 epinephrine, injected through a 25-gauge needle into the various standard portal sites (2–6 and midcarpal) down to the level of the capsule with or without intra-articular infiltration. Their standard setup consisted of placing a patient's arm on the metal base plate of the traction tower with the shoulder abducted, elbow flexed to 90°, forearm in neutral rotation, and the hand in an erected position with hand subjected to digital traction through the plastic finger traps. Apart from pain (average VAS score 3–5) there were no immediate complications.

SOME KEY POINTS IN APPLYING THIS TECHNIQUE TO WRIST AND SMALL JOINT ARTHROSCOPY

Surgeons who wish to perform the arthroscopy using WALANT technique should be proficient already with performing the procedure under general or regional anesthesia, because the WALANT procedure demands the most precise technique.

Intraoperative complications could occur and surgeons need to be aware of the added pressures that could come from an awake patient. This underlies the importance of having a good surgical team who not only understand the procedure but also could provide the necessary support to the surgeon as well as the patient. Surgeons who wish to adopt WALANT technique in their practice should be prepared to reschedule a procedure or convert to general anesthesia if it becomes necessary. These potential issues should be addressed during preoperative preparation and consent process.

The technique of administering local anesthetic has been refined with the development of portal site local anesthesia. In combination with dorsal capsule local anesthetic infiltration, effective anesthesia can be reliably achieved with only a small volume of local anesthetic, which then allows for accurate placement of portals in wrist arthroscopy. Apart from surgical proficiency and careful patient selection, the successful execution of wide-awake small joint arthroscopy relies on a meticulous preparation. Surgeons need to pay particular attention to the positioning, setup, availability of appropriate equipment, timing of local anesthesia, and skill level of the scrub team.

Arthroscopy has been used increasingly in treating wrist or distal radioulnar joint discorders.[10–12] With further popularity of minimal invasive approaches and local anesthesia in hand surgeons,[13–20] the authors believe that this technique will be extended to the arthroscopy of the wrist and small joints of the hand by more hand surgeons. The authors have found wide-wake wrist or small joint arthroscopy a reliable and satisfactory procedure. Patients who underwent this procedure were able to view their internal articular anatomy and engage with an on-table discussion about the relevant findings and treatment. This reinforces patients' confidence in the surgeons and encourages patients to comply with postoperative rehabilitation.

SUMMARY

The advent of wide-awake arthroscopy has given surgeons the ability to visualize both static and dynamic movements of a joint and to assess dynamically a surgical procedure that has been performed, which may help to avoid future postoperative problems. With increased familiarity with WALANT technique and improved technology of arthroscopic instruments, the spectrum of procedures that can be safely performed inside small joints using the wide-awake technique are expected to rise. Most excitingly, the novel extended application of d-WAWA has provided new insight in the assessment of carpal instability and has also challenged current understanding of carpal kinetics.

REFERENCES

1. Ho PC, Lo WN, Hung LK. Arthroscopic resection of volar ganglion of the wrist: a new technique. Arthroscopy 2003;19:218–21.
2. Ong MTY, Ho PC, Wong CWY, et al. Wrist arthroscopy under portal site local anesthesia (PSLA) without tourniquet. J Wrist Surg 2012;1:149–52.
3. Hagert E, Lalonde D. Wide-awake wrist arthroscopy and open TFCC repair. J Wrist Surg 2012;1:55–60.
4. Mak MCK, Ho PC, Tse WL, et al. Arthroscopic resection of wrist ganglion arising from the lunotriquetral joint. J Wrist Surg 2013;2:355–8.
5. Geissler WB, Freeland AE, Savoie FH, et al. Intracarpal soft-tissue lesions associated with an intra-articular fracture of the distal end of the radius. J Bone Joint Surg Am 1996;78:357–65.
6. Berger RA. A technique for arthroscopic evaluation of the first carpometacarpal joint. J Hand Surg Am 1997;22:1077–80.
7. Walsh EF, Akelman E, Fleming BC, et al. Thumb carpometacarpal arthroscopy: a topographic, anatomic study of the thenar portal. J Hand Surg Am 2005;30:373–9.
8. Slutsky DJ. The use of a dorsal-distal portal in trapeziometacarpal arthroscopy. Arthroscopy 2007;23:1244.e1-4.
9. Koo SJJ, Ho PC. Wrist arthroscopy under portal site local anesthesia without tourniquet and sedation. Hand Clin 2017;33:585–91.
10. Mathoulin CL. Indications, techniques, and outcomes of arthroscopic repair of scapholunate ligament and triangular fibrocartilage complex. J Hand Surg Eur Vol 2017;42:551–66.
11. Luchetti R, Atzei A. Arthroscopic assisted tendon reconstruction for triangular fibrocartilage complex irreparable tears. J Hand Surg Eur Vol 2017;42:346–51.
12. Nakamura T, Abe K, Nishiwaki M, et al. Medium- to long-term outcomes of anatomical reconstruction of the radioulnar ligament to the ulnar fovea. J Hand Surg Eur Vol 2017;42:352–6.
13. Lalonde DH. Conceptual origins, current practice, and views of wide awake hand surgery. J Hand Surg Eur Vol 2017;42:886–95.
14. Gong KT, Xing SG. How to establish and standardize wide-awake hand surgery: experience from China. J Hand Surg Eur Vol 2017;42:868–70.
15. Tang JB, Gong KT, Zhu L, et al. Performing hand surgery under local anesthesia without a tourniquet in China. Hand Clin 2017;33:415–24.
16. Lalonde D, Bell M, Benoit P, et al. A multicenter prospective study of 3,110 consecutive cases of elective epinephrine use in the fingers and hand: the Dalhousie Project clinical phase. J Hand Surg Am 2005;30:1061–7.
17. Wong J, Lin CH, Chang NJ, et al. Digital revascularization and replantation using the wide-awake hand surgery technique. J Hand Surg Eur Vol 2017;42:621–5.
18. Lalonde D. Minimally invasive anesthesia in wide awake hand surgery. Hand Clin 2014;30:1–6.
19. Gregory S, Lalonde DH, Fung Leung LT. Minimally invasive finger fracture management: wide-awake closed reduction, K-wire fixation, and early protected movement. Hand Clin 2014;30:7–15.
20. Lalonde D, Eaton C, Amadio P, et al. Wide-awake hand and wrist surgery: a new horizon in outpatient surgery. Instr Course Lect 2015;64:249–59.

Wide Awake Surgery as an Opportunity to Enhance Clinical Research

Verena J.M.M. Festen-Schrier, MD[a,b],
Peter C. Amadio, MD[a,*]

KEYWORDS

• Tendon • Muscle • Nerve • Physiology • Human

KEY POINTS

- Wide awake surgery allows the clinician-scientist to observe and measure active function of muscle tendon units before, during, and after surgical intervention. In addition to improving clinical results empirically, this capability allows novel expansions of physiologic research previously not possible in humans.
- Wide awake-enhanced research can improve the ability to correlate muscle function and physiology with clinical outcome after procedures such as tendon transfers, and correlate muscle and tendon forces with clinical activities such as pinch and grip.
- Wide awake-enhanced research has the potential to improve the understanding of the correlation between nerve physiology and motor and sensory function.

By now we are becoming more familiarized with the Wide Awake Local Anesthesia No Tourniquet or the WALANT technique, and its accompanying advantages. From a clinical perspective, the limitations as a result of general anesthesia are lifted, relieving patients from strict presurgical instructions and assessments, possible accompanying side effects, an intravenous line, and a hospital stay. However, the advantages of WALANT are not limited to the clinical experience alone. In this article, the authors describe potential new areas and opportunities for research by using different research-related aspects and placing them within the context of the WALANT approach to hand surgery.

EXTENSION OF OPERATION TIME AND INTRAOPERATIVE MOTION ASSESSMENT

Depending on the location and extent of the surgical procedure, different total volumes and concentrations of injectate can be used to acquire the desired effect, varying from 1% lidocaine and 1:100,000 epinephrine to 0.25% lidocaine and 1:400,000 epinephrine.[1] This results in up to 2.5 hours of effective local anesthesia without the need for a tourniquet; even for longer procedures the main limitation is patient fatigue and difficulty in remaining still for extended periods of time, as dosing can be repeated, even if longer-acting anesthetics are not used. This elongated window of opportunity allows for the clinical researcher to make full use of another beneficial feature of WALANT versus general anesthesia: the ability to have the patient actively move their wrist, hand, or fingers allows for direct physiologic measurements that would otherwise have been either obtained indirectly by imaging modalities or not possible at all. Because hand anatomic dimensions are highly individualistic, any nonindividual estimates are hard to generalize, which emphasizes the added

Disclosure Statement: The authors have no financial interest to declare in relation to the content of this article.
[a] Department of Orthopedic Surgery, Mayo Clinic, 200 First Street Southwest, Rochester, MN 55905, USA;
[b] Department of Plastic, Reconstructive and Hand Surgery, Erasmus Medical Center, Rotterdam, The Netherlands
* Corresponding author.
E-mail address: pamadio@mayo.edu

Hand Clin 35 (2019) 93–96
https://doi.org/10.1016/j.hcl.2018.08.003

value for research outcomes of intraoperative patient specific assessments.

Wide awake hand surgery by itself is not new, and research studies have used the advantages of wide awake surgery for years, albeit through a much shorter time window due to the historical avoidance of the use of epinephrine in the hand, for reasons now discredited,[1] with the need to complete studies before tourniquet pain and tourniquet-induced paralysis drawing the investigation to a conclusion. Within these restrictions, researchers in the past were able to quantify tendon forces in order to better understand normal digit function. One such study, for example, measured flexor tendon forces during carpal tunnel release surgery.[2] Using an S-shaped buckle transducer, tendon forces were measured during a set of different active motions and correlated with fingertip load. This required the patient's full cooperation during surgery, but could be accomplished within a 10- to 15-minute window. Similar studies could, for example, correlate tendon, nerve, and synovial motion after carpal tunnel release, as a novel way to quantitate the effect of adhesions on motion, and to validate noninvasive ultrasound measurements.

Wide awake surgery has also been described as a means to test surgical repair success, to test the need for adjustment of tendon tension before closure of the skin, and to test the patient's cognitive adaptation to tendon transfers.[3] One study observed that all patients (n = 7) could extend their thumb immediately after the commonly performed extensor indicis proprius to extensor pollicis longus tendon transfer, without any special education. Based on these results, the investigators concluded that the concept of formal reeducation after tendon transfer in the hand may require reevaluation, and that it is more likely that a preexistent neural system is recruited to cope with the new alignment. This opens an exciting new field of research whereby other procedures and the ability of the patient's adjustment to a new "wiring" construction can be assessed within a very short timeframe through the use of WALANT.

Intraoperative measurement of muscle properties has been described by Lieber and colleagues.[4–6] Sarcomere length has a significant impact on force generation in a muscle and should therefore affect surgical results. However, it is extremely difficult to measure sarcomere length in living humans for research purposes, for one due to the need of tissue exposure.[7] In addition, results of tendon transfer in particular can be very surgeon and clinical situation dependent, making generalization and the design of specific guidelines challenging.[8] WALANT allows for intraoperative

measurements with laser diffraction techniques[4,5] to quantify sarcomere overlap, indicating the achievement of a stage of muscle resting length at the end of the surgical procedure. Simultaneous comparison of these measurements with theoretic modeling has already been shown to be a powerful tool to help the surgeon better predict functional outcomes.[6] With WALANT, because of the increased operating time permitted, further refinements are also possible. A hypothesized model combining tension of the transfer, intraoperative force during pinch or grip, and sarcomere length and all of their correlations could now, for example, be measured to address scientific questions related to optimal functioning of the tendon transfer. Research questions concerning the presence of, if any, a functional disadvantage of setting the transfer slightly tighter than physiologic length of the muscle could also be tested. With physiologic length accurately assessed by sarcomere length, and with the ability under WALANT to measure many aspects of hand function in the operating room, and even to change them, such questions can be answered empirically.

IMAGING VALIDATION

Part of developing novel imaging techniques or data analysis protocols is the necessity to establish both the repeatability and the validity of the technique. The first meaning that similar results are acquired when performing the same type of measurement on the same subject multiple times, and the latter indicating that any quantitative measurements provided by the imaging modality adequately reflect physiologic truth. Validation is more often done using either cadaveric samples or phantom models, which in their own respect can approximate the clinical situation but also have intrinsic limitations. For example, in the context of carpal tunnel syndrome (CTS), many studies have used B-mode ultrasound imaging in order to improve the accuracy of diagnosis or to help predict treatment outcome.[9,10] More recently, dynamic imaging of tendon and nerve motion, as well as movement of the surrounding synovium (which is thickened in CTS and also distinctly visible ultrasonographically), has been added to the repertoire.[11–13] WALANT-based research can, for example, explore the hypothesis that stiffening of the connective tissue around the carpal tunnel structures might underlie part of the CTS pathophysiology.[14] Although part of the validation work for a particular displacement analysis technique called speckle tracking has been done in cadavers[15] and phantoms,[16] a real-time validation could also be done using a wide awake approach during live surgery.[17] The latter of course best represents the clinical situation in which the clinician would later incorporate the imaging method. Dissociation between the movement of flexor tendons and the covering visceral synovium has also been documented in vivo during carpal tunnel release surgery.[18]

SEPARATING THE EFFECT ON FUNCTION OF A SURGICAL PROCEDURE VERSUS HEALING

During any type of anatomy-altering procedures (as compared with fixation type surgeries), the hand surgeon can use the patient's ability to actively move to assess the effect of the procedure based on the mechanical properties of the subjected structures and those that surround them. Although this type of immediate feedback is indispensable for surgeons to review their work, it has the limitation of only providing the expected result if mechanics were the only influencing factors. However, after surgery, patient activity postoperatively and wound healing also impact the result noted in follow-up. The WALANT approach allows for a baseline assessment of the patient's strength, range of motion, and other functions first before, and then after, all surgical interventions have been completed, while the patient is pain free but fully awake and with strength unimpeded by sedation or paralysis. These measurements in turn serve as the true baselines against which any subsequent measurements can be made, before any postoperative changes have occurred. This in turn allows the researcher as well as the clinician to distinguish the immediate mechanical change of the procedure from the subsequent biological effects on functionality. In addition, the intraoperative measurements can be correlated with final outcome, to determine whether factors such as strength or excursion predict the final outcome.

LOGISTICAL ADVANTAGES IN RESEARCH

Not having the necessity to have to do the surgery under general or regional anesthesia not only allows more logistical freedom in terms of planning and staffing, but also increases the total time available for research and opens up opportunities to add elements that could not have been used otherwise. This is particularly true if WALANT is done in the office setting. Examples of the logistical advantages would be the assessment of the desired outcomes (eg, function, patient survey, MRI) immediately before the surgery or the opportunity to more easily bring in medical imaging devices for intraoperative correlations. The surgical procedure will still need to be done within a sterile

field, but the addition of, for instance, a sterilized ultrasound probe is much easier to achieve, especially with imaging modalities becoming increasingly more mobile and smaller.

From a research perspective, it is always important to respect and minimize the impact and burden on the patient/research subject. Decreasing the patient's logistical load could help in lowering the participation threshold without a negative effect on data acquisition. In addition, it comes with a decreased risk involved with the procedure, due to the safer form of anesthesia, allowing for a complementary expression of beneficent action. Clinical research is almost fully done on a voluntary basis and thus depends on the willingness of subjects to spend their time and energy by getting involved in studies. Any changes that lower the threshold for participation would therefore directly benefit the course of a study. Being able to communicate with a patient throughout the procedure adds another helpful element: Getting patients to successfully engage in research is highly dependent on their personal interest and emotional link to the research topic and potential outcomes,[19] and an extra moment of conversation could go a long way in achieving that level of involvement, just as it does in helping the patient better understand the procedure and the postoperative care. In addition, potential costs associated with a study can be minimized by simplifying the surgical environment, providing more opportunities not only in developed countries but also in less developed low- and middle-income countries.

Decreased costs will also be helpful in any type of research in which trainees play a role. Training surgical residents is an investment in time, effort, and monetary expense,[20] which can be particularly challenging when working within a research budget. Expanding the repertoire of office-based procedures through the use of WALANT can be very helpful in this context. Not having to use a full operating room and being less limited in time due to the absence of a tourniquet means that residents can be more actively involved in the surgical procedure if allowed in the research context. Second, using training aspects as a main topic of investigation (eg, comparison of different teaching strategies) is possible, to study not only resident education but also the intraoperative patient education strategies that might positively affect outcome.

RESEARCH ABOUT WIDE AWAKE SURGERY UNDER LOCAL ANESTHESIA WITH NO TOURNIQUET ITSELF

Of course, WALANT can not only facilitate physiologic and other clinical research based on the procedures that can be performed using WALANT. WALANT can itself be the subject of research. WALANT dramatically reduces intraoperative bleeding: does this result in less postoperative inflammation, less pain, and better healing? Such hypotheses can be tested. As noted above, intraoperative education can also be studied, to identify the features most likely to improve patient outcomes.

SUMMARY

To conclude, the combination of advantages provided by the WALANT technique is valuable, not only from a clinical point of view but also when viewed from a research perspective. WALANT-facilitated and WALANT-focused research both open new horizons for study, not possible previously. As WALANT becomes more widely adopted at academic centers, such opportunities will be more often grasped. Indeed, the scholarly opportunities offered by WALANT present a strong argument for the adoption and dissemination of WALANT.

REFERENCES

1. Lalonde DH. Conceptual origins, current practice, and views of wide awake hand surgery. J Hand Surg Eur Vol 2017;42:886–95.
2. Schuind F, Garcia-Elias M, Cooney WP, et al. Flexor tendon forces: in vivo measurements. J Hand Surg Am 1992;17:291–8.
3. Bezuhly M, Sparkes GL, Higgins A, et al. Immediate thumb extension following extensor indicis proprius-to-extensor pollicis longus tendon transfer using the wide-awake approach. Plast Reconstr Surg 2007; 119:1507–12.
4. Lieber RL, Loren GJ, Fridén J. In vivo measurement of human wrist extensor muscle sarcomere length changes. J Neurophysiol 1994;71:874–81.
5. Lieber RL, Yeh Y, Baskin RJ. Sarcomere length determination using laser diffraction. Effect of beam and fiber diameter. Biophys J 1984;45: 1007–16.
6. Lieber RL, Fridén J. Intraoperative measurement and biomechanical modeling of the flexor carpi ulnaris-to-extensor carpi radialis longus tendon transfer. J Biomech Eng 1997;119:386–91.
7. Son J, Indresano A, Sheppard K, et al. Intraoperative and biomechanical studies of human vastus lateralis and vastus medialis sarcomere length operating range. J Biomech 2018;67:91–7.
8. Murray WM, Hentz VR, Fridén J, et al. Variability in surgical technique for brachioradialis tendon transfer. Evidence and implications. J Bone Joint Surg Am 2006;88:2009–16.
9. Fowler JR, Gaughan JP, Ilyas AM. The sensitivity and specificity of ultrasound for the diagnosis of carpal tunnel syndrome: a meta-analysis. Clin Orthop Relat Res 2011;469:1089–94.
10. McDonagh C, Alexander M, Kane D. The role of ultrasound in the diagnosis and management of carpal tunnel syndrome: a new paradigm. Rheumatology (Oxford) 2015;54:9–19.
11. Kuo T-T, Lee M-R, Liao Y-Y, et al. Assessment of median nerve mobility by ultrasound dynamic imaging for diagnosing carpal tunnel syndrome. PLoS One 2016;11(1):e0147051.
12. van Doesburg MHM, Henderson J, Mink van der Molen AB, et al. Transverse plane tendon and median nerve motion in the carpal tunnel: ultrasound comparison of carpal tunnel syndrome patients and healthy volunteers. PLoS One 2012;7(5): e37081.
13. Wang Y, Filius A, Zhao C, et al. Altered median nerve deformation and transverse displacement during wrist movement in patients with carpal tunnel syndrome. Acad Radiol 2014;21:472–80.
14. Werthel J-D, Zhao C, An K-N, et al. Carpal tunnel syndrome pathophysiology: role of subsynovial connective tissue. J Wrist Surg 2014;03:220–6.
15. Korstanje J-WH, Selles RW, Stam HJ, et al. Development and validation of ultrasound speckle tracking to quantify tendon displacement. J Biomech 2010; 43:1373–9.
16. Revell J, Mirmehdi M, McNally D. Computer vision elastography: speckle adaptive motion estimation for elastography using ultrasound sequences. IEEE Trans Med Imaging 2005;24:755–66.
17. Stegman KJ, Djurickovic S, Dechev N. In vivo estimation of flexor digitorum superficialis tendon displacement with speckle tracking on 2-d ultrasound images using laplacian, gaussian and rayleigh techniques. Ultrasound Med Biol 2014;40: 568–82.
18. Ettema AM, Zhao C, Amadio PC, et al. Gliding characteristics of flexor tendon and tenosynovium in carpal tunnel syndrome: a pilot study. Clin Anat 2007; 20:292–9.
19. Bartlett SJ, Barnes T, McIvor RA. Integrating patients into meaningful real-world research. Ann Am Thorac Soc 2014;11(Supplement 2):S112–7.
20. Allen RW, Pruitt M, Taaffe KM. Effect of Resident involvement on operative time and operating room staffing costs. J Surg Educ 2016;73:979–85.

Extending Applications of Local Anesthesia Without Tourniquet to Flap Harvest and Transfer in the Hand

Shu Guo Xing, MD*, Jin Bo Tang, MD

KEYWORDS

- Flap • Anesthesia • Tourniquet • Wide-awake hand surgery • WALANT

KEY POINTS

- Flap harvest and transfer in the hand can be performed under local anesthesia with epinephrine. This procedure is another example of the broadening applications of wide-awake surgery. The authors' experience demonstrates that wide-awake flap surgery in the hand is safe.
- The authors used the wide-awake local anesthesia no tourniquet approach in 4 commonly used flaps in the hand: the extended Segmuller flap, the homo-digital reverse digital artery flap, the dorsal metacarpal artery perforator flap, and the Atasoy advancement flap.
- Wide-awake flap surgery works very well and safely achieved excellent anesthetic and vasoconstrictive effects in the authors' cases.
- The authors have found that vasoconstriction caused by epinephrine mainly affects the capillaries. It does not affect digital arteries and their major branches in the hand. The authors found that harvesting a flap in the hand and fingers may not be a contraindication to wide-awake surgery.
- An approach of injection of epinephrine with lidocaine 15 minutes before flap harvest, and injection of phentolamine immediately after flap transfer may be universally and routinely applied to most microvascular surgical procedures, including digital artery–based pedicled flaps or perforator flaps in the hand.

INTRODUCTION

It is generally considered that epinephrine should not be used in combination with microvascular surgery or any vessel-related surgery in the hand. Flap surgery was thought to be a contraindication because of the vasoconstrictive effects of epinephrine, but there is a lack of evidence to support this.[1–7] In fact, the authors have found that local anesthetic with epinephrine in the hand in microvascular dissection and flap harvest is possible and safe.

Based on the transient vasoconstrictive effects of epinephrine on the vasculature of only capillaries, the authors think that it is possible to use epinephrine and local anesthetic for flap harvest and transfer. The authors think that soft tissue flaps will not suffer avascular necrosis in 4 to 5 hours because they can routinely successfully perform digital replantation after 6 to 8 hours of ischemia. This article reviews the authors' experience of flap harvest and transfer in 27 flap transfers in the fingers and hand.

METHODS OF LOCAL ANESTHESIA INJECTION

The authors used 1% lidocaine with 1:100,000 epinephrine buffered with 8.4% sodium

Department of Hand Surgery, The Hand Surgery Research Center, Affiliated Hospital of Nantong University, 20 West Temple Road, Nantong 226001, Jiangsu, China
* Corresponding author.
E-mail address: xingshuguo10@163.com

Hand Clin 35 (2019) 97–102
https://doi.org/10.1016/j.hcl.2018.08.009
0749-0712/19/© 2018 Elsevier Inc. All rights reserved.

bicarbonate in a 10:1 ratio.[8] In their patients, the average volume infiltrated into each digital ray was 19 mL. The authors injected most of it at the level of the distal palmar crease to minimize the effect of compression on the vessels in the finger itself.[9,10] The following describes the method of local anesthesia with epinephrine injection for each of 4 flaps.

Extended Segmuller Flap

The mean volume of local anesthetic infiltration administered is about 19 mL per digital ray for harvesting this flap (**Fig. 1**A). First, about 10 mL is injected volar to the level of metacarpophalangeal (MP) joint. This injection at the base of the finger acts as a temporary sympathetic block in the finger distal to the injection that may help prevent vasospasm.[11] Hyperemia in the finger distal to the white epinephrine at the digit base makes this evident. The anesthesia of this injection also helps the authors remove the wound dressings without pain. After waiting about 5 minutes, the authors inject another 2 mL, 2 mL, and 1 mL under volar finger skin at the level of the MP, proximal interphalangeal, and distal interphalangeal (DIP) joint creases, respectively. Finally, they inject 2 mL and 2 mL in each of the dorsal central aspects of the proximal and middle phalanges, respectively.

Homo-Digital Reverse Digital Artery Flap

The injection method is the same as for an extended Segmuller flap.

Atasoy Flap

The authors inject about 11 mL per digital ray for this flap (**Fig. 1**B). First, about 10 mL is injected volar to the level of the MP joint. After waiting for about 5 minutes, the authors inject 1 mL at the level of the DIP joint crease distally.

Dorsal Metacarpal Artery Perforator Flap

The authors inject about 20 mL to harvest this flap (**Fig. 1**C). First, about 10 mL is injected proximal to the designed flap. After waiting for 5 minutes, they inject 5 mL and 5 mL to the central and metacarpal head parts of the flap. They are careful to inject beside the likely location of the flap perforator, not right in the perforator. They do not want to damage the perforator with the needle. Then they inject no more than 9 or 10 mL in the area between the defect and the flap.

Waiting Time Between Injection and Surgery

After the injection of the lidocaine and epinephrine, the authors typically wait only 15 minutes to start flap dissection. They have found that there is no need to wait for 20 to 30 minutes to begin surgery in these patents. During these 15 minutes, they perform preoperative preparation by cleansing the skin and draping the area.

POSTOPERATIVE CARE

After the surgery, trained nursing staff monitor all the authors' patients every 30 minutes for 5 hours until the flap is well perfused for digital artery–based pedicle flaps or perforator flaps but only for 30 minutes after harvesting an Atasoy flap. If critical flap ischemia is been encountered, the authors have phentolamine (1 mg diluted in 1–10 mL saline) available to reverse the vasoconstrictive effects of epinephrine. However, the authors injected phentolamine only once in the whole series. It was during the surgery for the one patient who had a *dorsal metacarpal artery perforator flap* to help verify its vascular supply. The flap pinked up nicely and quickly. This injection was the only time that the authors used phentolamine in their series. They did not need to inject phentolamine after surgery in any of their 27 patients.

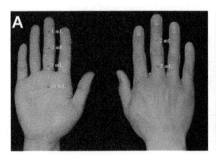
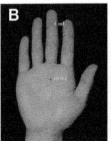
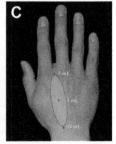

Fig. 1. Injection of local anesthesia. (*A*) The point (*red dot*) and volume of injection for extended Segmuller flap and homo-digital reverse digital artery flap. (*B*) The point and volume of injection for Atasoy flap (advancement flap). (*C*) The points and volume of injection for the dorsal metacarpal artery perforator flap.

THE AUTHORS' PATIENTS

From April 2017 to March 2018 the authors used the aforementioned anesthesia method in 27 fingers (age range 18–67 years old) for flap harvest and transfer after traumatic defects of fingertips as well as dorsal and central finger wounds. The authors did not apply this method to patients with

- Unilateral or bilateral digital bundle injuries (recent or previous)
- A history of a peripheral vascular disorder
- Considerable procedural anxiety who preferred intravenous sedation or brachial plexus block anesthesia

Table 1 summarizes the use of the 4 flaps in the authors' 27 patients. All of the authors' flaps were performed by experienced hand surgeons.[12] After debridement of devitalized tissues, the flaps were harvested using the previously described techniques.[13–17]

Observation of Blood Supply to Flaps

The authors did not use digital or other tourniquets to aid in the identification and dissection of structures. At the time of the skin incisions, they noted some bleeding; but, as they reached the deep tissues, the bleeding decreased and the field was clear enough to allow the procedure. All the cases had adequate bleeding control (**Figs. 2** and **3**). The authors could clearly see digital arteries pulsate even though they were bathed with 1:100,000 epinephrine (**Fig. 4**).

No patient required phentolamine for digit or flap ischemia during or after surgery except the one with the dorsal metacarpal artery perforator flap transfer as described earlier. That patient had a pale flap during surgery. A total of 10 mL of phentolamine was prepared by diluting 1 mg phentolamine into 10 mL saline. The authors injected 4 mL into the flap after flap elevation: 1 mL of phentolamine to the proximal, middle, and distal parts, respectively, and 1 mL near the pedicle of the flap without injuring the perforator. The authors supplemented injection to the sites where they found fluid leakage. The flap pinked up and survived completely.

Pain and Satisfaction

No patients required termination of the procedure because of pain. Overall, 96% of patients (26 of 27) stated that they would have the procedures performed under wide-awake local anesthesia no tourniquet (WALANT) if they had to have the procedure again. Only one patient stated that he would not choose WALANT again because of anxiety during surgery.

Postoperative Flap Survival and Complications

The survival of the flaps of these patients was monitored for a mean of 14 days (range 8–16 days). All flaps except for one survived completely without overt venous congestion or ischemia. Early in the authors' series, one patient having an extended Segmuller flap had partial necrosis in a 3-mm strip of skin at the very distal part of the flap. It healed without further surgery. This strip was less than 5% of the flap. This complication may have been attributed to too much tension on the distal edge of the skin flap after skin closure. No patient sustained a syncopal event. One patient had superficial infection that resolved with oral antibiotics.

SAFETY OF FLAP SURGERY WITH WIDE-AWAKE LOCAL ANESTHESIA NO TOURNIQUET

The use of epinephrine in microvascular surgery has been discouraged because of possible skin ischemia or infarction, which theoretically may be caused by epinephrine vasoconstriction with the WALANT technique. However, with the many benefits of WALANT surgery and the continuing evolutions of its application, the authors have questioned whether or not the theoretic contraindication to epinephrine is valid in real life.

Table 1 Summary of the number of patients using 4 different flaps			
Flaps	**Numbers**	**Intraoperative Findings**	**Phentolamine**
Extended Segmuller flap	9	Good blood supply	No
Homo-digital reverse digital artery flap	3	Good blood supply	No
Atasoy flap (advancement flap)	14	Good blood supply	No
Dorsal metacarpal artery perforator flap	1	Poor blood supply	Intraoperative injection needed

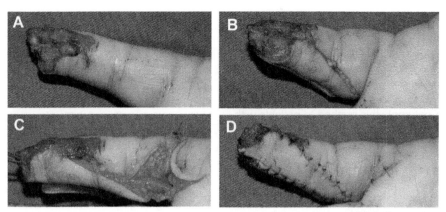

Fig. 2. The extended Segmuller flap harvest and transfer for a defect in the fingertip of the left little finger under local anesthesia with epinephrine. (*A*) The area of defect was 2.1 × 1.6 cm. (*B*) The flap was harvested from the radial side of the finger with good perfusion. (*C*) The pulsatile digital artery–based flap was advanced to the recipient site. (*D*) The appearance of the flap after operation.

Epinephrine causes constriction of capillaries, not the larger vessels, such as digital arteries. The authors could see the digital arteries pulsate despite being bathed with 1:100,000 epinephrine. They, therefore, now know it is safe to harvest digital artery–based flaps when epinephrine is used. The perforator-based flap may be more vulnerable to the vasoconstrictive effect of epinephrine. In the authors' one patient with the dorsal metacarpal artery perforator flap, they injected phentolamine to reverse the epinephrine vasoconstrictive effect at the time of surgery. That flap pinked up and completely survived after phentolamine injection.

The effect of epinephrine usually only lasts for 4 to 5 hours. It only causes *incomplete* ischemia of vasoconstricted tissues. Typically, incomplete ischemia of a flap for 4 to 5 hours does not lead to necrosis.

Wong and colleagues[18] have shown it is possible to safely and successfully perform digital replantations and revascularizations using WALANT. They showed that anastomosis of digital arteries and veins in the hand under local anesthesia with epinephrine is feasible, because the vasoconstriction caused by epinephrine mainly affects the capillaries. This finding helped the authors be confident that the transient vasoconstrictive effects of epinephrine could be used safely in flap harvest and transfer and emergency patients.[19,20]

LIMITATIONS

The limitations of WALANT for hand flap surgery include that it is difficult to assess flap perfusion with capillary refill or skin color because of the vasoconstrictive action of epinephrine. However, the authors have only used it in pedicled or advancement flaps, so such an observation is not critically necessary. In the authors' patients, none had flap loss. The authors have found that the blood supply of the flap usually recovered after 4 to 5 hours after the epinephrine injection. If the blood supply of the flaps cannot be determined, the authors can inject phentolamine for reversal of vasoconstriction during the operation, as they did in the one patient with dorsal metacarpal artery perforator flap.[21,22]

Fear of use this approach to microsurgery still exists, even in the authors' unit, where wide-awake surgery is routine for all hand surgeons. It is a new extension of the technique. Only one of the authors' teams of hand surgeons has attempted this technique; but the authors think that this report will stimulate others to help them define its application and points of attention before, during, and after surgery.

SUGGESTED APPROACHES

Should surgeons want to monitor blood perfusion of the skin or worry about the effect of epinephrine,

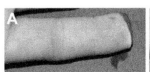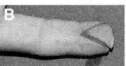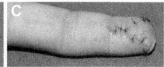

Fig. 3. Atasoy flap (advancement flap) was applied in a 41-year-old woman under local anesthesia with epinephrine. (*A*) The defect area was 1.3 × 1.2 cm. (*B*) Atasoy flap design and skin incision. (*C*) The flap is moving distally to cover the defect with adequate perfusion.

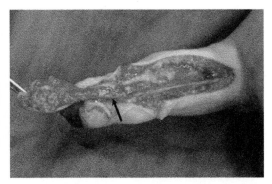

Fig. 4. The pulsations in the digital artery (*black arrow*) were easily observed during the wide-awake homo-digital reverse digital artery flap surgery, even though the artery was bathed with 1:100,000 epinephrine.

they could inject phentolamine *immediately* after surgery as a routine in all patients who have this anesthesia. Although the authors did not have to inject except in one patient, they consider that such an approach of *injection of epinephrine with lidocaine 15 minutes before flap harvest, and injection of phentolamine immediately after flap transfer* may be universally applied to most microvascular surgical procedures, including digital artery–based pedicled flaps or perforator flaps harvested in the hand. The Atasoy flap and Moberg flaps, which are more traditional local flaps, are even safer for using epinephrine with lidocaine, without any need of phentolamine. We also consider it proper to use epinephrine in the finger or thumb when the tip needs artificial dermal templates.[23] However, we suggest avoiding epinephrine when amputation is treated with a composite graft without anastomosis of the vessels.[24]

SUMMARY

The authors present their techniques of hand and finger flap harvest and results in 27 patients. The flaps were all harvested under local anesthesia with epinephrine without a tourniquet. All flaps had good perfusion to the flap by 4 to 5 hours after the operation. One flap had a successful injection of phentolamine to reverse the effect of epinephrine during the surgery. The authors propose the approach of *injection of epinephrine with lidocaine 15 minutes before flap harvest, and injection of phentolamine immediately after flap transfer* for hesitating hand surgeons. This approach may be universally and routinely applicable to most microvascular surgical procedures, including digital artery–based pedicled flaps or perforator flaps in the hand. More traditional local flaps, such as Atasoy or Moberg flaps, are very safe for using epinephrine with lidocaine, without the need of phentolamine.

REFERENCES

1. Lalonde DH. Reconstruction of the hand with wide awake surgery. Clin Plast Surg 2011;38:761–9.
2. Xing SG, Tang JB. Surgical treatment, hardware removal, and the wide-awake approach for metacarpal fractures. Clin Plast Surg 2014;41: 463–80.
3. Tang JB, Gong KT, Zhu L, et al. Performing hand surgery under local anesthesia without a tourniquet in china. Hand Clin 2017;33:415–24.
4. Gong KT, Xing SG. How to establish and standardize wide-awake hand surgery: experience from China. J Hand Surg Eur Vol 2017;42:868–70.
5. Steiner MM, Calandruccio JH. Use of wide-awake local anesthesia no tourniquet in hand and wrist surgery. Orthop Clin North Am 2018;49:63–8.
6. Lalonde DH. Conceptual origins, current practice, and views of wide awake hand surgery. J Hand Surg Eur Vol 2017;42:886–95.
7. Rhee PC, Fischer MM, Rhee LS, et al. Cost savings and patient experiences of a clinic-Based, wide-awake hand surgery program at a military medical center: a critical analysis of the first 100 procedures. J Hand Surg Am 2017;42:e139–47.
8. Lalonde DH, Wong A. Dosage of local anesthesia in wide awake hand surgery. J Hand Surg Am 2013;38: 2025–8.
9. Lalonde D. Minimally invasive anesthesia in wide awake hand surgery. Hand Clin 2014;30:1–6.
10. Prasetyono TO. Tourniquet-free hand surgery using the one-per-mil tumescent technique. Arch Plast Surg 2013;40:129–33.
11. Chandran GJ, Chung B, Lalonde J, et al. The hyperthermic effect of a distal volar forearm nerve block: a possible treatment of acute digital frostbite injuries? Plast Reconstr Surg 2010;126:946–50.
12. Tang JB, Giddins G. Why and how to report surgeons levels of expertise. J Hand Surg Eur Vol 2016;41:365–6.
13. Venkataswami R, Subramanian N. Oblique triangular flap: a new method for oblique amputations of the fingertip and thumb. Plast Reconstr Surg 1980;66: 296.
14. Germann G, Rudolf KD, Levin SL, et al. Fingertip and thumb tip wounds: changing algorithms for sensation, aesthetics, and function. J Hand Surg Am 2017;42:274–84.
15. Tang JB, Landín L, Cavadas PC, et al. Unique techniques or approaches in microvascular and microlymphatic surgery. Clin Plast Surg 2017;44:403–14.
16. Usami S, Kawahara S, Yamaguchi Y, et al. Homodigital artery flap reconstruction for fingertip amputation: a comparative study of the oblique triangular neurovascular advancement flap and the reverse digital artery island flap. J Hand Surg Eur Vol 2015;40:291–7.

17. Tang JB, Elliot D, Adani R, et al. Repair and reconstruction of thumb and finger tip injuries: a global view. Clin Plast Surg 2014;41:325–59.

18. Wong J, Lin CH, Chang NJ, et al. Digital revascularization and replantation using the wide-awake hand surgery technique. J Hand Surg Eur Vol 2017;42:621–5.

19. Xing SG, Mao T. The use of local anaesthesia with epinephrine in the harvest and transfer of an extended Segmuller flap in the fingers. J Hand Surg Eur 2018;43:783–4.

20. Xing SG, Mao T. Temporary tourniquet use after epinephrine injection to expedite wide awake emergency hand surgeries. J Hand Surg Eur 2018;43:888–9.

21. Nodwell T, Lalonde D. How long does it take phentolamine to reverse adrenaline-induced vasoconstriction in the finger and hand? A prospective, randomized, blinded study: the Dalhousie project experimental phase. Can J Plast Surg 2003;11:187–90.

22. Zhu AF, Hood BR, Morris MS, et al. Delayed-onset digital ischemia after Local anesthetic with epinephrine injection requiring phentolamine reversal. J Hand Surg Am 2017;42:479.

23. Elliot D, Adani R, Woo SH, et al. Repair of soft tissue defects in finger, thumb and forearm: less invasive methods with similar outcomes. J Hand Surg Eur Vol 2018;43:1019–29.

24. Eo S, Doh G, Lim S, et al. Analysis of the risk factors that determine composite graft survival for fingertip amputation. J Hand Surg Eur Vol 2018;43:1030–5.

Moving?

Make sure your subscription moves with you!

To notify us of your new address, find your **Clinics Account Number** (located on your mailing label above your name), and contact customer service at:

Email: journalscustomerservice-usa@elsevier.com

800-654-2452 (subscribers in the U.S. & Canada)
314-447-8871 (subscribers outside of the U.S. & Canada)

Fax number: 314-447-8029

**Elsevier Health Sciences Division
Subscription Customer Service
3251 Riverport Lane
Maryland Heights, MO 63043**

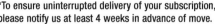

*To ensure uninterrupted delivery of your subscription, please notify us at least 4 weeks in advance of move.

Printed and bound by CPI Group (UK) Ltd, Croydon, CR0 4YY

03/10/2024

01040301-0016